YOU CAN LOOK BETTER!

So many "vital statistics," such as age, social status, sex appeal, and likability, are judged on the basis of how you look. And your skin—its texture, color, and quality—is the most telling part of the picture.

So, if you can visualize yourself having the gently flushed skin of Renoir's bathers, this book was written for you!

YOUR SKIN

A DERMATOLOGIST'S GUIDE TO A LIFETIME OF BEAUTY AND HEALTH

FREDRIC HABERMAN, M.D. AND DENISE FORTINO

BERKLEY BOOKS, NEW YORK

YOUR SKIN: A DERMATOLOGIST'S GUIDE
TO A LIFETIME OF BEAUTY AND HEALTH

A Berkley Book / published by arrangement with
the authors

PRINTING HISTORY
PBJ Books edition / January 1983
Berkley edition / April 1983
Fourth printing / March 1986

ISBN: 0-425-09589-4

A BERKLEY BOOK ® TM 757,375
Berkley Books are published by The Berkley Publishing Group,
200 Madison Avenue, New York, NY 10016.
The name "BERKLEY" and the stylized "B" with design
are trademarks belonging to Berkley Publishing Corporation.

PRINTED IN THE UNITED STATES OF AMERICA

Dedicated with love and gratitude to
Harvey and the late Sylvia Haberman,
Ernest and Claire Fortino

ACKNOWLEDGMENTS

The authors would like to thank Barbara Pipines and Susan Allen for their invaluable help throughout the writing of this book. Our gratitude also to Michael Haberman, M.D., Atlanta-based psychiatrist and Clinical Assistant Professor of Psychiatry at Emory University, for his gracious assistance and thoughtful contributions to the sections on the psychology of skin disorders; as well as to Sarah Uman and Linda Healey, our editors; Sheila, Renée, and Elisa Haberman, Dominick D'Alleva, Diana Benzaia, Bryna Gilgor and all our other close relatives and friends for their unfailing patience and support.

Special thanks to Robert S. Gilgor, M.D., associate professor of medicine (dermatology), division of dermatology, department of medicine, Duke University Medical Center, Durham, North Carolina, and associate professor of medicine (dermatology) at the University of North Carolina School of Medicine (Chapel Hill), whose dedication and excellence in the field inspired Dr. Haberman to pursue a specialty in dermatology and give it his "all-out effort."

Finally, the following physicians have been involved in Dr. Haberman's training and continuing medical education as a dermatologist: Michael Fisher, M.D., professor of medicine, Albert Einstein College of Medicine, director, dermatology division, Bronx Municipal Hospital Center and Hospital of Albert Einstein College of Medicine, New York City; Peter Burk, M.D., associate professor of medicine (dermatology) Albert Einstein College of Medicine, and chairman, division of dermatology, Montefiore Hospital, New York City; Gerald S. Lazarus, M.D., former associate professor of medicine (dermatology) Albert Einstein College of Medicine and former chairman, division of dermatology, Montefiore Hospital, New York City, now professor and chairman, department of dermatology, School of Medicine, University of Pennsylvania; Lowell Goldsmith, M.D., former professor of medicine (dermatology), Duke University Medical Center, now professor and chairman, department of medicine (dermatology), University of Rochester School of Medicine.

The material on Eczema and Hives, as well as the quizzes on Acne and Dermatitis have been provided by Robert S. Gilgor, M.D., of the Duke University Medical School, North Carolina.

Contents

CHAPTER 1

KNOW YOUR SKIN

Skin at its best is easy to describe: supple, smooth, exquisitely elastic, blemish-free; with a clarity often compared to the sheerness and refinement of porcelain. It is the tender, touchable flesh of babies, the gently flushed bodies of Renoir's bathers, the finely contoured complexions of high-fashion models. To most people, staying young means preserving this flawless, fresh-faced look forever. Yet so many resign themselves to changes they consider inevitable, especially during adolescence and middle age. The fact is that most of us can enjoy magnificent skin throughout our life in return for some surprisingly simple efforts. The body's largest organ is also its most resilient and responsive to daily care.

Of course, since the skin is the only organ on public display (except when tucked under clothes or masks!), even its minor malfunctions may seem momentous. One oddly placed pimple can spell agony before a date or business meeting. Someone who has avoided doctors for years may rush off to a dermatologist at the very first sign of troubled skin.

Quite literally, your skin is all that lies between you and the outside world. Yet it is not just decorative wrapping; no other part of the body is more versatile or complex. Knowing something of its "inside" story can help you keep it in the best of shape. Only by being well informed will you be able to head off potential problems on your own and obtain the most dramatic results from any outside treatment, should you require it.

Your Remarkable Skin

If it were stretched out flat (and it is very stretchable), your skin would cover an area of roughly two square yards, and weigh about eight pounds. A relentless vigilante, it shields you from the environment's hostile elements (pollutants, chemicals, bacteria), releases internal impurities yet prevents loss of precious fluids, cushions and insulates vital organs, and protects from extremes of heat and cold. Naturally waterproof, skin will not allow liquids past its topmost layers, so you can never become bloated while you bathe or swim. While it keeps your insides in and holds you firmly in place, this amazingly durable material also allows great flexibility and ease of movement. Like a well-made balloon, it is capable of expanding and contracting as parts of the body swell or diminish in size.

Think of skin, too, as one massive erogenous zone. Attuned to the ebb and flow of hormones, it receives and relays the signals of sexual arousal—tactile, visual, emotional. Its intricate network of nerves can register the heights of physical pleasure and warn against the subtlest pressure and pain. It tells you when you are being stroked or squeezed, distinguishes damp from dry and burlap from cotton, and can even detect the faintest breeze.

While it contains all that you are, skin also reveals your

condition with uncanny accuracy. A yellow, ashen, or blotchy complexion is often a first alert that something elsewhere is amiss. Even serious disorders, including diabetes, thyroid problems, and liver disease, may announce their arrival through telltale changes on the surface. Simple tension, fatigue, a faulty diet, too little fresh air and exercise, and repeated self-neglect can all leave their unflattering marks as well.

Omnipresent and inescapable, skin is always being manipulated in some way—rubbed, kneaded, scratched, pulled, or picked; chilled, or heated; adorned, painted; steamed, burned, or weathered by the elements. Whether decorated or damaged, it heartily survives these myriad shocks and stresses of everyday living.

The reason: Your "miracle" skin is continually renewing and replacing itself. This makes it one of the most remarkable organs of the body, as most others, once formed, remain unchanged. The outer portion, or epidermis, about as thick as a page of this book, consists of about fifteen to twenty layers of closely connected cells, which near the surface overlap like roof shingles. Those in the basal, or bottommost, layer are forever dividing and pushing their way toward the surface—the hardened "protective shell" called the stratum corneum. As the plump newborn cells make their ascent, they gradually flatten out, lose moisture, cast off their inner mainspring (nucleus), and eventually die. Normally an upwardly mobile cell takes about two weeks to reach its destination and another one or two to be shed or sloughed away. Washing, rubbing, and ordinary wear and tear help this process steadily along. (When this mechanism goes awry and cells are shed too rapidly, disorders such as psoriasis and dandruff may result.)

Scattered throughout the basal layer are branch-shaped cells called melanocytes. These manufacture granules of melanin, a natural brown-black pigment that gives skin its characteristic tone and color. (Everyone, regardless of race or sex, has the same number of melanocytes; heredity determines the size of the granules and the amount of pigment they produce.) Melanin is yet another natural shield. When exposed to sunlight, the skin protects itself by simply churning out more melanin, a process known as tanning. The pigment granules absorb ultraviolet radiation, which can severely damage living cells. However, since a tan is only a partial protection at best, a sunscreen is necessary to complete the defense. (See Chapter 7.)

Deeper down lies the tough, fibrous, remarkably elastic *dermis,* which derives its shape and strength primarily from collagen, the protein known as "nature's nylon." The sweat and oil glands, blood vessels, and nerves all play out their endless drama here.

Like a spiraled ball of twine, each sweat gland has a free end, which winds its way up to the epidermis. As many as two to five million of these microscopic coils are embedded in human skin. Every day they secrete about one and a half pints of a clear, alkaline mixture mostly composed of water, urea, and salts. When carried to the surface, the fluid evaporates, taking heat from the body and cooling it down—a kind of natural thermostat. Physical exertion, excessive heat, emotional stress, anxiety, alcohol, even certain foods or medications, stimulate the glands to greater activity.

The body's temperature is also regulated by a vast network of dermal capillaries. Responding to outside conditions, these expand or contract, either to release or to conserve heat from circulating blood. They also deliver vital nutrients and oxygen to the epidermal cells above. And these diminutive vessels impart color to the skin as well. You blush red when they dilate, turn "white" when they constrict.

Another group of residents of this layer, the sebaceous glands, which cluster chiefly on the face, neck, and back, release an oil that spreads out on the surface of the skin and serves as a natural moisturizer. Along with fluids from the sweat glands, this softens and lubricates the dried-up outer cells, guards against erosion by dust and wind, and keeps the surface slightly acid to discourage harmful bacteria from taking root. Harsh soaps, detergents, and chemicals can help strip away this natural protective mantle, leaving the skin more susceptible to chapping and infection.

The third and deepest layer of skin is the subcutaneous layer, or underlying fatty tissue. Composed mostly of stored fat cells, connective tissue, and strands of collagen, it serves as a shock absorber, heat retainer, and nutritional reservoir. It also provides a passage for nerves and blood vessels, as well as some deeply penetrating hair follicles and sweat glands. This resilient layer is considerably more ample in women, imparting a typically fine-spun texture to their surface skin.

To be successful, any treatment for beautiful skin must consider all its crucial components—the protective upper cells and the nourishing, supporting tissues. How fast you age visibly depends more on how you care for your total skin, both outer and inner layers, and on your general health than on your chronological age.

To sum up the secrets of lifelong youth: Keep sun exposure to a minimum, since the sun damages collagen and hastens wrinkling and drying more than any other single factor. Eat sensibly—a wholesome variety of fresh, unadulterated foods—to keep skin tissues well nourished, blood flowing smoothly, and all glands and nerves in peak working order. Get adequate rest and recreation, and curtail habits such as smoking and hard drinking, which can discolor skin on the surface and undermine it underneath.

Cleanliness is another secret to youthful, glowing skin—but this does not mean scrubbing away with great volumes of soap, which can clog pores and strip away natural oils. Moisturizing should also be part of the daily regimen for certain skins, and here, too, striking a healthful balance is essential for best results. Choose natural cloths over synthetic materials, which can trap excess moisture instead of letting it flow and evaporate normally. And beware of systemic medications such as cortisone and estrogens, which can wreak havoc in the form of blemishes and damage capillaries.

Genetic makeup (for example, whether you are fair-haired or thick-skinned), lifestyle, work environment, climate (warm, steamy weather tends to breed acne), and emotional health also help determine the state of your skin. In the pages that follow, you'll discover how and why these factors play such a prominent role and how to keep the equation in your favor.

Skin and Psyche

So many "vital statistics," such as age, social status, sex appeal, and likability, are judged on the basis of how you look. And skin—its texture, color, and quality—is the most telling part of that picture. Looking at the face alone may uncover some remarkably personal details, both physical and psychological. Possible alcohol or drug abuse, age, internal diseases, fluctuations in weight, vanities, tastes, indiosyncrasies, and personality traits may all be available for inspection by the casual observer!

The cells of the brain and skin originate from the same tissue as an embryo develops, so it is not difficult to see how the two can be intimately related. Emotions in all their subtle and dramatic variations are almost instantaneously reflected in the face. You may pale and sweat with anxiety and fear, and flush with excitement or embarrassment. You can actually see how a person feels—whether he is depressed, fatigued, tense, or elated and self-confident—by looking at his skin.

Not surprisingly, emotional turmoil may underlie a host

of skin disorders. Acne, hives, and eczema, for example, can be triggered or intensified by nervous tensions at work or by the anger that smolders after a quarrel at home. A self-inflicted syndrome called *lichens simplex chronicus* arises from simple repetitive nervous scratching, which results in severely irritated, thickened, even ulcerated skin. Why? When people are anxious or preoccupied, they often perspire more profusely, and the added surface moisture can lead to an itch/scratch/itch cycle that eventually becomes automatic. Scratching itself, even in the absence of discomfort, can turn into a habitual, mindless way of releasing anxiety. Another ''nervous habit'' problem is *trichotillomania*, the partial hair loss that results from relentlessly pulling and twisting the hair. Hairs are short, stubbly, and of varying lengths, and the bald patches are shaped irregularly (which distinguishes the condition from the hair loss caused by disease).

People who are acutely sensitive about their appearance in general and about their skin in particular will often compulsively squeeze and pick at their acne or other blemishes, however imperceptible these may be. This behavior could represent an unconscious desire to punish themselves for being less than perfect or to erase the damaging evidence. In the process, however, they only succeed in driving the lesions deeper into the skin and increasing the risk of permanent scarring.

Why do some of us respond to stress by developing skin disorders (or by becoming obsessed with our skin), while others protest the assault with ulcers or migraine headaches? Scientists are not absolutely sure, although they suspect that genes play a role in how the body handles stress. Thus, emotional factors alone may not cause troubled skin unless you are already genetically programmed for that response.

Learned behavior also can account for different ways of expressing anxiety or channeling nervous tension. Thus, some chain-smoke through a crisis, while others doodle feverishly or chew on nails. When you respond to stress by hurting yourself in some way, underlying guilt or self-destructive impulses may be at work. For example, a number of people have great difficulty voicing any anger or hostility, especially in the presence of authority figures or loved ones. So they may learn to suppress "forbidden" feelings by clenching and grinding their teeth or pulling and tugging at their skin, as if turning the unacknowledged anger back on themselves.

Psychiatrists are fond of saying—and the pun is quite intentional—that people who habitually scratch their face or body have "things that get under their skin." Hard-driven, Type A perfectionists, demanding of both themselves and others, are well represented among this group. For such people, hypnosis and/or short-term psychotherapy can be very effective cures. Once they confront the source of their anxiety and find a healthier outlet for pent-up feelings, the skin disorder generally clears.

Those whose jobs do not allow for the easy expression of dissatisfactions and complaints are also prime candidates for such psychosomatic problems. Often the victims of self-inflicted damage to the skin are plagued by other tension-related disorders as well: acid stomach, elevated blood pressure, possible dependence on mood-altering drugs or alcohol. At certain stages of life—adolescence, midlife, after graduation or embarking on a new career, during the early years of a marriage—we are all more susceptible.

Stress usually acts on the skin indirectly, via the neuro-endocrine system, which involves both the nerves and the glands. Many skin disorders can be traced to infections, allergies, or hormone imbalances, and chronic stress may be at the root of all three. For example, the levels of thyroid adrenaline, steroids, and sex hormones in your body are subject to fluctuations in emotions and moods. Since these natural chemical messengers collectively influence skin color, tone, elasticity, oil gland activity, circulation, hair growth, and new cell production, any radical change among them can have a telling impact on the way you look.

When the body is under stress, it often responds by releasing more androgens (male hormones), present in both men and women. These in turn activate the oil glands, and the frequent result is acne. At any age acne can be psychologically disabling. At puberty, when you are especially concerned about putting your best face forward, biology can deal a very cruel blow by enlarging and stimulating the same troublemaking glands.

Striving for independence and acceptance by peers, coping with new bodily sensations, an awakening sexual identity, and a developing sense of self can all make this a particularly confusing, explosive time. If an adolescent's family sets rigidly high standards for achievement or inhibits the fullest expression of feelings and fears, he or she may respond by withdrawing emotionally. A blackhead or blemish may seem an imperfection that threatens less love and acceptance from parents and friends; compulsive picking to make it disappear is one way of coping with such a threat.

In their quest for reflected glory, some parents perpetuate adolescent insecurity by pressuring their children to excel in every way, including the way they look. They may unwittingly damage self-esteem by making insensitive comments about pimples, hair, noses, and other obvious targets. Sometimes a parent harbors an ideal, or mental plan, of a child's life and appearance. If that image includes perfect physical features, severe acne and other skin disorders can lead to disappointment and injured pride. Such parental disapproval, even if only subtly and obliquely expressed, can be picked up by any vulnerable adolescent. Unfortunately, emotional difficulties caused or aggravated by skin problems at any age may have far-reaching consequences for the rest of a person's life.

Obsession or Reality?

A condition called narcissistic personality disorder is being diagnosed by an increasing number of psychiatrists these days. To oversimplify, people with this problem continually seek approval and assurance of self-worth by measuring up to some elusive external standard, such as physical perfection. They feel undeserving and undesirable unless they look impeccable or project a perfect image. However, by vainly pursuing an abstraction, an impossible ideal, they doom themselves to chronic dissatisfaction and become vulnerable to even the slightest changes wrought by time. Every new wrinkle, graying hair, or pound of added weight may become a source of panic. Their continual self-absorption also makes it difficult for them to relate lovingly or easily to others.

Psychiatrists agree that someone obsessed with physical appearance is probably playing out a more deep-seated insecurity. Thus, an otherwise attractive person may experience intense anxiety over a minor facial flaw, while another, far less good-looking, will enjoy buoyant self-confidence. As psychiatrist Dr. David D. Burns observes in his book, *Feeling Good: The New Mood Therapy* (William Morrow/Signet), "A poor self-image is the magnifying glass that can transform a trivial mistake or an imperfection into an overwhelming symbol of personal defeat." In such cases, in which a person seizes on a physical feature to express a general discontent, psychotherapy may be necessary to expose the underlying problem.

However, even with your self-esteem intact, you may

still suffer hangups and inhibitions if you are convinced that all is not right with your skin or some other part of your body. These feelings can subtly or even profoundly affect the way you relate to others, and are not altered if people disagree or call you overly modest about your appearance. Regardless of how you really look, as long as you *feel* unattractive, your body confidence will diminish. Even worse, others will pick up your negative signals and will probably shy away, thus reinforcing your own self-doubts. Often just improving or correcting that single blemish on your body-image, whether real or exaggerated, can help you feel immeasurably better about yourself. In turn, these positive personal vibrations will more readily attract both friends and lovers, since confidence is undeniably contagious.

It is not unusual for the person with newly cleared skin to seek a total makeover. A change of wardrobe and hairstyle, along with a renewed interest in dieting and exercise, often follows the successful treatment of a skin disorder.

One high school student, overweight and plagued with acne, expressed her unhappiness and disgust with herself by generally avoiding close contact with members of both sexes. After her skin was successfully treated, however, she felt motivated enough to lose weight—a goal that had eluded her for years—and the rebound effect happily continued. Next she restyled her hair, decided to run for student council, and began "coming out" socially. Having clear skin alone did not automatically grant her self-acceptance, but it was a powerful psychological boost that helped her emerge from hiding and reverse her negative body image.

Obviously skin is such a central aspect of ourselves that we are likely to celebrate and complement its health and beauty by enhancing ourselves in other ways as well. When it does not look its best, our impulse is to hide; we feel drained of morale and motivation, inclined to let ourselves go.

Fortunately the vast majority of skin problems respond readily to treatment and can be prevented with proper care. The aging process can be slowed down by the right precautions and a variety of recently refined techniques, and even possibly reversed. And the skin has its own capacity to repair and regenerate itself.

Once you have identified your individual "skinprint" and evaluated your skin's special needs, you will be on your way to the beautiful, healthy face and body you have always wanted—and you will have them for a lifetime.

CHAPTER 2

FIND YOUR SKIN TYPE

From the newborn black baby's to that of the Scandinavian octogenarian, all human skin shares the same superbly structured form and function, though there are a number of variations on the common theme. Some skin types are acne-prone, for example, while others are susceptible to chafing or highly sensitive to the sun. Still others tend to wrinkle or sag at an earlier than usual age.

Is your complexion dry, oily, extra fragile, just plain normal, or some unique combination of these? Find which description roughly matches yours in the brief guidelines that follow. By pinpointing your skin's special strengths and weaknesses, you will be able to take better care of it. But do not assume that any verdict is final. Your skin's characteristics may vary according to changes in season, age, environment, and even emotional needs.

Dry Skin
Feels taut, spiny, and rough after washing and is likely to develop dry surface lines, or pseudo-wrinkles, especially around the cheeks, eyes, and mouth. Often fairly thin, transparent, and/or fine-textured with hardly visible pores. Can appear flaky and cracked, with a dull, matte finish, and may chap or redden easily when exposed to strong winds or cold. Rarely breaks out.

Normal Skin
A relatively rare condition! The surface is flexible, smooth, firm, and even-textured, neither flaky nor slippery to the touch either before or after washing. Pores are hardly visible, and a good oil/moisture balance keeps breakouts, if any, short-lived and minimal. Normal skin often tans more readily than it burns. The color is natural, and the complexion looks clear, fresh, and well scrubbed.

Oily Skin
May feel sticky, clammy, and unclean because of excess surface oils. Texture can be coarse and thick, pores large and visible, and complexion often has an ashen or sallow cast. Tends to tan easily. The forehead and chin sport a telltale shine sometimes only an hour or two after the face is washed or makeup applied. Acne is common, often persistent.

Combination Skin
Perhaps the most common variety of all. As the name suggests, this kind of skin is dual: oily along the so-called T-zone (forehead, nose, and chin), complete with visible pores and breakouts; dry, flaky, and sensitive to wind and sun around cheeks, eyes, and mouth.

Sensitive or Allergy-Prone Skin
Any type of skin may also belong in this category. Easily chafed by wool; harsh soaps, abrasive detergents, rough washcloths make it feel tender, burning, irritated. Blood vessels may dilate after consumption of hot, spicy foods, coffee, or alcohol. Blotching, hives, itching, swelling, or worse may result after contact with proven irritants such as strawberries, lanolin, or formaldehyde. Those with black skin should be extra vigilant, since irritation or inflamma-

tion from any source can cause noticeable, sometimes permanent, changes in pigment.

As the above descriptions suggest, one easy way to judge your skin is to use the sun as a gauge. If you burn readily, your skin is usually drier and needs more protection from the elements, especially a good moisturizer, than one that tans easily. The light eyes/fair hair/freckles combination is one extreme, while dark eyes, hair, and skin is another. Everything else falls in between.

Be aware that within each type, skin conditions can vary widely. For example, very oily skin may be marked by especially persistent or inflammatory acne and seborrhea, abnormally dry skin by cracking around the lips or exceptional susceptibility to infection. The extremes may require a dermatologist's care, though the suggestions that follow should help temper even the severest symptoms.

Thorough cleansing regimens for all skin types are covered in Chapter 9; the guidelines below include such steps as moisturizing and toning, along with general directions on how and when to wash.

Daily Strategies

For Dry Skin
After washing in the morning with a mild soap in lukewarm water, rinse thoroughly and blot dry with a soft towel. While skin is still damp, apply a cream-type moisturizer such as Nivea or Eurecin. Use a cream- or oil-based

foundation and blusher. In the evening, a sterile absorbent-cotton pad soaked first in water then in a mild astringent, such as alcohol or witch hazel will remove last traces of makeup. Rinse, then wash gently and moisturize as you did in the morning.

About twice a week you might try an egg yolk and honey mask. Beat a small egg yolk, add a few drops of water and 1 tablespoon of honey. With fingers or a soft basting brush, apply to face, using a light upward, circular movement; spread over neck, using gentle downward strokes. Leave on for 10 or 15 minutes, then rinse gently with lukewarm water.

Alternate Tips: After cleansing and before moisturizing, apply a facial of equal parts of buttermilk and yogurt. Pat all over face, neck, and throat, avoiding the eye area. Let dry, then rinse with cool or tepid water. If skin is especially dry, allow buttermilk to stand at room temperature overnight and use the cream that rises to the top. (For more on facial masks, see Chapter 10.)

In winter, weather-proof skin with an extra layer of moisturizer before going outdoors.

Optional: Apply eye cream before bedtime.

Makeup Tips: For a fresh, dewy glow (to offset the mat look of dry skin), thin out any liquid foundation with a few drops of water and a dab of moisturizer. Or use the brush and buff technique: Apply translucent powder with a brush over foundation, then whisk the excess away with a slightly dampened sponge. (For more on how to apply makeup, see Chapter 10.)

For Oily Skin
After washing in the morning with a mild or gentle detergent soap in lukewarm water, rinse thoroughly and blot dry with a soft towel. Wet a ball of sterile absorbent cotton with astringent and rub it over your entire face, especially

forehead, nose, and chin, and include your hairline as well. (Astringents are more effective when kept chilled in the refrigerator.) Rinse face again in cool water and gently apply a light moisturizer, preferably a mild urea-based product such as Aquacare HP or U-Lactin, which will not block or irritate already oily pores. Blot any remaining lotion after spreading on a fine layer. Repeat the same ritual in the evening minus the moisturizer.

Use water-based or oil-free foundations and blushers.

Dust face and body with loose powder throughout the day and use pre-moistened towelettes to curb excess oils. (A shiny face accentuates oversized pores and facial creases.) If you do not have acne, you may include a loofah or Buf-Puf in your nighttime routine up to three times a week.

Or try an almond or oatmeal facial to slough away outer scaly cells. Mix a handful of rolled oats or ground almonds with warm water to make a thin paste. Apply to dampened skin, avoiding the eye and mouth areas. Leave on for 5 to 10 minutes, then wipe off gently with a wet washcloth. Rinse with warm running water.

Alternate Tips: To tone down an unwanted shine, stir a packet of active dry yeast into warm water to make a pastelike consistency. Spread on the face, leave for 10 minutes, then rinse. Or spread thinly sliced unpeeled cucumbers or potatoes on the face—especially bracing during summer. Or add a teaspoon of table salt to a spray bottle of water. Mist face with the mixture, then carefully rub off with a soft towel.

Shampoo frequently. Grimy hair adds extra oil to your face.

In summer change and wash sweatbands frequently if you are an active athlete or avoid them altogether; they are perfect grease-collectors, especially when worn for long periods of time. During hot, humid weather or after a strenuous exercise workout, step up your washing routine accordingly, but don't use harsh formulas that strip away protective natural oils. Take lukewarm showers. Avoid wearing makeup or lotions while exercising, especially in summer, and use gel-type (drying) sunscreens. Keep hair swept away from face or tied back during vigorous activity.

An occasional steaming may help loosen blackheads and draw out surface oils. Pour boiling water into a bowl or sink and add some chopped fresh herbs, such as chamomile or comfrey, if you like. Hold your face about 12 inches from the surface of the water for 5 to 10 minutes, draping a towel over head and bowl to trap the steam. Blot face dry with a soft towel.

Makeup Tips: To help set makeup or foundation and hold it longer before shine shows through, finish off with a light dusting of baby powder or talc powder. On a fresh-scrubbed face without makeup, they help keep shine away and soak up excess oil.

For Combination Skin

Morning and night follow directions for oily skin, but confine most vigorous cleansing to the T-zone area (forehead, nose, and chin). While skin is slightly damp, use moisturizer primarily on cheeks, near mouth, and on neck. Apply chilled astringent to the T-zone. You may try the masks for both dry and oily skin—just be sure to use them on the appropriate sections of your face. If you wish to steam occasionally, afterward be sure to use a moisturizer wherever skin is dry and an astringent on the oily parts.

For Normal Skin

Since this type has a good oil/moisture balance, almost any soap or moisturizer will do (twice a day), preferably gentle formulas, neither overly rich nor drying, designated for problem-free skin. Facial masks are rarely necessary, though these may be soothing during unusually dry or humid conditions.

Keep in mind that even the most balanced complexions begin to lose moisture with age, especially after forty. So as you grow older, start observing the routines that apply for dry skin. (See also Chapter 8.)

If you are in the twenty-five to thirty-five age group, the onset of dry patches for the first time may signal a change from normal or oily to combination skin. Since the outer edges of the face are now drier than the middle, these tend to chap and flake more noticeably after washing, especially if you are not used to a light-touch approach. The answer is to follow directions for combination skin, cleansing and moisturizing in a more selective way.

Even with gentle washing, dry, crusty patches can sometimes develop over normal or even chronically oily skin. One suspect is seborrhea, a form of facial dandruff triggered by overworked oil glands. If you mistake the condition for simple dryness, you may apply moisturizer to ease the roughness and scaling and wind up making matters worse. Seborrhea should be treated by a dermatologist. Occasionally eczema or psoriasis can cause such dry islands, complicating the condition with itching and inflammation. Both conditions require a doctor's care. (See also Chapter 12.)

For Sensitive Skin

Skin should be cleansed with very mild products no more than twice a day. Use soapless lotions such as Lowila and Keri Facial Cleanser or toilet soaps or natural vegetable-oil soaps made without detergents and scents. Stay away from obviously dyed, vividly colored bars. Always wash and rinse with tepid water and be sure to remove soapy films and makeups thoroughly. To minimize irritation from astringents, apply them with water-soaked sterile cotton pads.

Use makeup that has been formulated without potentially troublesome fragrances, oils, and preservatives. Buy it in small quantities and get fresh supplies periodically. Avoid prolonged exposure to cold or hot brisk wind and excessive sunlight. Besides a daily sunscreen, apply an extra coat of moisturizer before going out, especially when the weather is dry and blustery.

See also Chapter 10. Much of the information there on cosmetics and skin reactions applies to sensitive and allergy-prone skin.

A Guide for All Skins

Because of environmental conditions, both natural and man-made, dry, perennially thirsty skin is probably one of the most persistent problems of all. Dryness means a low level of moisture—water—so even people with oily skin and especially people with combination skin may have chronic trouble on certain parts of the face and body, particularly after overdoing it with soaps or astringents. Whenever you wash too frequently or vigorously, you strip your outer skin of its naturally protective mantle. Even an acne-studded face may feel taut, drawn, and flaky as a result of overzealous cleansing or overdrying medications. (If you have acne, a light, non-greasy moisturizer may help counterbalance skin-parching treatments.)

Partly because of how we adapt to them, the seasons can also be moisture-depleting. Skin, like a concrete road, will crack with sudden temperature changes, especially during the rigors of a freezing, thawing winter. Besides an oil-gland slowdown at this time of year, the combination of raw, brisk winds and overheated rooms makes winter an especially dehydrating season. During cold months, the average home has a humidity level as low as five to fifteen percent, a condition drier than either Death Valley or the Sahara Desert! Any atmosphere with a relative humidity lower than thirty percent will rob moisture from your skin. Remember, everyone marvels at the traditionally dewy complexions of the English, who live in a humid climate and for the most part do not have central heating.

When the surface of the skin is dry, chapped, or fissured, chemicals and bacteria can penetrate more easily, causing irritation or even infection. An overly dry interior can also clog the nasal passages, which results in breathing through the mouth. This, in turn, leads to tiny cracks in the lips. When people lick their lips to restore the moisture, they end up by making the chapping worse. Lip balms, moisturizing lipsticks, and sun protection sticks can counter dryness during all seasons and protect against ultraviolet damage as well.

To help guard against moisture loss indoors, check your insulation. When warm air is dissipated through a poorly insulated roof or leaking doors and windows, moisture steadily evaporates. To combat the problem, burn fewer fires, keep the fireplace flue closed as much as possible, and fix the thermostat so low that no family member will be tempted to open a window. Other skin-saving investments are humidity gauges, motor-driven humidifiers (for homes with forced-air heat), and moisture-recycling electric (not gas) clothes dryers that can be vented within. Buy at least a bedroom-size or cold-water humidifier. To prevent mold and mildew use fungicidal or mold control tablets regularly. Cold-water humidifiers should be cleaned with Lysol frequently, rinsed thoroughly, and allowed to dry.

Cultivate an indoor garden. Certain house plants can be skin-soothing treatments, filling the environment with moisture and a healthy supply of oxygen. Selecting the right kind of plant is crucial, since many draw more water from the air than they release and so have a dehydrating effect on skin. Choose types that are happiest with wet feet, that require plenty of water and are fast growers. The best indoor varieties are bamboo, most ferns (especially the maiden-hair family), large-leafed plants such as begonias (not the waxed kind, however), zebra plant, coleus, spathiphyllum, and papyrus.

The potted plants should be placed in a wide, shallow tray filled with pebbles or moss and water. This keeps the air around the leaves well saturated, allowing the plants to release the maximum moisture. The soil should be constantly damp and the leaves misted often. Giving such actively metabolizing, water-drinking plants this extra-humid environment allows them to work their hardest to keep your skin healthy.

Another natural way to humidify the air is to leave a few inches of water in the bathtub or sink. Drape a towel over the side of the tub so that the end is submerged, making it a natural wick. Place an attractive, water-filled bowl on each radiator. An eight-quart pot placed over a simmering flame will release about five or six gallons of water during a twenty-four-hour period.

Keep yourself lubricated inside, too, by drinking a lot of water, especially in air-conditioned or overheated rooms.

Avoid laundering with enzyme detergents, powdered bleaches, and whiteners. During winter use only one-fourth the amount of detergent the manufacturers suggest. Tattletale gray sheets are better than chafed, lobster-red skin. But even gently laundered clothing worn too tightly, especially wools and nylons, can constrict circulation and irritate already dehydrated skin. If skin is very irritated or inflamed, short-term use of a prescription steroid cream may be a solution. (Prolonged application can intensify dryness.)

Even at your oiliest, do not overwash with soaps, astringents, abrasive washcloths, pore-minimizers, grains, or loofahs. Above all, do not linger in the bathtub and soak for an hour or take long showers. Paradoxically, the longer the skin is exposed to water, the more the dead cells of the stratum corneum absorb and the more they will shrink when they dry out, paving the way for a classic case of thirsty skin.

In summer, air conditioning, chlorine, salt water, extra showers, and air travel in pressurized cabins are all notorious skin-dehydrators. Of course, the effect of air conditioning should be the reverse of that of steam and forced-air heat. But most systems strip away too much moisture in the mechanical cooling process, leaving the chilled air with less humidity than the original warm atmosphere.

Moisturizing: How and Why

Besides watching the thermostat and taking steps to conserve humidity, the best way to stave off dryness all the year round is by the proper use of a moisturizer. The principle at work is very simple. You have heard that oil and water do not mix, but both are indispensable to moisturizers. Water is continually drawn upward through the layers of skin to the surface, where it evaporates. If water is lost at a faster rate than it is replenished, the skin feels dry and uncomfortable. When there is enough fluid in the outer cells of the epidermis, the skin swells, or plumps up slightly and becomes smooth and flexible. Sebum, produced by the oil glands, is a natural barrier against moisture loss, but it is often insufficient as you age or in an overly dry environment. The job of a moisturizer is to supplement sebum, to seal in the skin's fluids with a light film of oil.

The best time to apply moisturizer is after washing or bathing and toweling off only lightly, when the skin surface is still slightly damp, so that added moisture as well as the skin's own supply is retained for maximum effect.

Regardless of their ingredients, moisturizers are basically oil in water. (Technically they are called emulsions, which means that one or more substances have been added to make the oil and water hold together without separating.) Those with more water than oil are lotions; when oils predominate, creams are the result. Generally lotions are appropriate for oily skin, creams for dry, although conditions indoors or out may dictate a change of rule. For example, as the relative humidity rises in summer, your skin will lose less moisture to the air. This means that you may be able to switch to a lighter product if you spend more time outdoors than in drying, air-conditioned rooms.

Some moisturizers are deliberately designed to duplicate the skin's natural chemistry. For example, urea and lactic acid, present in skin sweat, are leading ingredients in many products, including Aquacare HP, Lacticare, Paraben, and U-Lactin. These are best for oily, normal, and combination skins, since they are relatively light, greaseless, and non-clogging.

Heavier bases such as lanolin and petrolatum, found in such products as Nivea cream, Vaseline petroleum jelly, Aquaphor, and Eucerin, are the most penetrating and longest-lasting moisturizers. Experiments have shown that they go on working to lubricate skin and retain moisture weeks after they have been discontinued. These are ideal for very dry skins, though a small percentage of people are allergic to raw lanolin. Greasiness can be minimized by dusting face and body with talc or baby powder after applying moisturizer. Substances such as isoprophyl myristate, isopropyl palmitate, stearic acid, and glyceryl stearate cut the oiliness of lanolin and petrolatum, resulting in a more elegant product. However, if used excessively, these ingredients are also potent irritants, which can trigger acne.

Mineral oil, hydrophilic ointment (which attracts watèr especially well), and squalene (derived from shark-liver oil and also found in human skin) are also highly effective moisturizers. Other products, boasting more extravagant claims and higher prices, are packed with such nourishing and reassuringly natural items as whole eggs, milk, and collagen. But there is no evidence whatever that these soothe dry skin any better or faster.

Black Skin

Black skin can be dry, oily, or somewhere between, and it also poses some special problems of its own. Blacks have the same number of pigment-producing cells as Caucasians; the difference is that in black skin each of the melanin granules they churn out is large and completely filled with color, whereas the granules in white skin are relatively small and separated from one another, packed in little membrane-covered bundles.

Since melanin provides a natural barrier or shield against damaging ultraviolet rays, the advantages of extra pigment are a much lower incidence of skin cancer and fewer facial wrinkles. But the quality that makes black skin more resistant to the ravages of time and sun also leaves it more vulnerable to other conditions. Thus, because pigment is so plentiful (and volatile), any injury, inflammation, or infection, from a minor cut or insect bite to surgery or severe acne, may result in a perceptible lightening or darkening of the skin. With acne, the problem can be compounded by using strong, abrasive medications, scrubbing with harsh soaps, and picking or squeezing.

In black skin, itching, inflammatory skin diseases, such as eczema and contact dermatitis (see Chapter 12), can result in a condition called pityriasis alba (light patches and scales) or in lichenification (clusters of tiny dark papules, triggered by friction and scratching, which join to form thickened plaques).

Raised, smooth, irregularly outlined blemishes, popularly called flesh moles, and darker than surrounding skin, may increase in size with age. White markings (hypomelanosis) are often found in older black skin, just like their equally harmless opposites, liver spots in white skin.

Excess pigment can be lightened with bleaching creams containing hydroquinone. Faded spots can be treated with special drugs and carefully timed doses of ultraviolet light (in order to activate melanin) or covered with a darker cream foundation until pigment returns. Of course, to obtain lasting results any source of irritation must be removed.

Following trauma or infection, ear-piercing, and occasionally acne, black skin is also more likely to develop thick raised scars called keloids. These stubborn flaws are overgrowths; they are larger than the wound that gave rise to them. Freezing with liquid nitrogen or injections of corticosteroids can reduce their size dramatically. Alternatively they can be surgically excised, then injected, leaving a smaller, more manageable scar in their place.

Overheated rooms, overwashing, and exposure to parching winds can lead to a buildup of dull, scaly outer cells, making black skin appear markedly gray or ashen. The best preventives are mild soaps, moisturizers, and room humidifiers.

Another black-skin problem, mostly affecting men, results from an inflammation of the hair follicles. Since the hair is naturally curved, even at the root, it sometimes has a tendency to curl back on itself, over the chin and scalp and reenter the skin. The ingrown hairs can form bumps, called pseudofolliculitis barbe, over the area of the beard. The bumps can fill with pus and become inflamed, a condition aggravated by shaving. Problem areas are the chin, jaw, and neck.

For some men a solution is to grow a beard and force the hairs to pop out again. Those for whom this is impractical are advised to shave not too closely and preferably every other day. For best results, before using the razor, apply a mixture of Vaseline and shaving cream to the beard with a toothbrusb, keeping with the grain, so to straighten out the hairs. Barbers' clippers or a motor-driven Oster finisher (an electric razor by Norelco designed especially for black skin) work best. Both do a thorough job quickly without exerting too much pressure.

Treat pus-filled areas with warm-water or saline compresses (1 teaspoon of salt to 1 pint of water) or Burrows soaks to reduce facial swelling. Oral or topical antibiotics can help if infection has set in, while remaining ingrown hairs can be rooted out with a sterile needle. (Never pull or pluck them or you will risk inflaming the hair follicles even more.)

Remember, black skin can be dry, normal, combination, oily, or extra-sensitive, so the same guidelines apply to black skin and lighter skin. But whatever the type or texture, always steer clear of soaps, astringents, and medications that are too abrasive. Overdrying and irritation can mar a black complexion all too visibly.

CHAPTER 3

ACNE: INSIDE AND OUT

> . . . and his cheeks were rivuleted and . . . eroded
> with acne. Among the old scars new pustules formed,
> purple and red, some rising and some waning. The
> skin was shiny with the medicines that were sold for
> this condition and which do no good whatever. . . .
> His mind and his emotions were like his face,
> constantly erupting, constantly raw and irritated. . . .*
> —John Steinbeck's description of Pimples Carson in
> *The Wayward Bus*

Freshly showered, her hair stylishly cut, Michele could
be wearing her best clothes and newest shoes yet still feel
dirty and unkempt. She recalls, "I always associated pimples with unwashed, scruffy people who never took care of
themselves. And I had gotten through adolescence without
more than an isolated blemish or two. Now, here I was at
eighteen, a good student, a responsible person, with a
faceful!"

She had watched her acne progress from a few easy-to-
hide red marks around forehead and chin to huge, unsightly cysts. "I grew bangs and sat in class with my
hands against my face just so nobody would notice. At

---

*As quoted also by W. J. Cunliffe, M.D., and J. A. Cotterill, M.D.,
in *The Acnes: Clinical Features, Pathogenesis and Treatment*.

home, I'd hold up mirrors at every angle to make sure my cosmetics had concealed them all. I could never rush out of the house on the spur of the moment to meet a friend. I'd always need at least fifteen minutes to play the cover-up game.''

All her tricks—longer hair, cupping her chin in her hand, heavy makeup—only made matters worse. And she found store-bought lotions and cleansers either too irritating or completely ineffective. In her case, even a doctor's care was no guarantee of success. "Few took the time to ask me about my daily habits or feelings, to test my skin type or sensitivity to certain medications, or to tell me what to expect from a given treatment. I accumulated a bagful of bottles in my search for the right physician.''

Some drugs were not given enough chance to work before she was switched to something else. Others were continued long after it was obvious that they were not doing the job. "A few doctors used mechanical extractors or curettes to remove my most obvious pimples. But since my dark skin pigments very easily, I was left with some equally noticeable scars and splotches in their place.''

The scarring proved more than skin deep. "If someone were attracted to me, I'd ask myself, 'What's wrong with him? How can he like me?—I have acne.' If I went for a job interview, I'd always imagine people shaking their heads and whispering, 'See that girl? She's so pleasant and well qualified. If only she didn't have such terrible skin!' Sometimes I'd pretend to be sick and would stay home from school if I had a particularly bad outbreak that morning. My acne worries even gave me a chronic upset stomach.

"And today, although my face is finally clear, I often act as if the acne still remains. The little leftover marks and craters may be barely visible to others, but to me they're huge and very obvious, a record of my shameful past. I'm not sure I'll ever be able to go out again without carefully applying makeup and checking mirrors first, even to mail a letter or wash the car. I am so used to hiding my imperfections, even though they no longer exist!''

Acne is by far our most universal skin disorder, affecting some seventy to nearly ninety percent of us at one time or other. It is also the oldest on record. The ancient Egyptian Ebers Papyrus, dating from 1500 B.C., bears a graphic description of the disease, and among the treasures entombed with the young King Tut were an assortment of acne remedies.

The condition takes a variety of forms, from a few scattered blackheads to deeply embedded cysts. But the familiarity of the problem is what makes it so invisible. Most people regard acne as an inescapable badge of puberty, a necessary rite of passage, rather than a disorder that calls for prompt attention. They may resign themselves to years of recurring outbreaks while waiting for the pimples to disappear on their own.

While few adolescents get by without at least some minor blemish, acne is not just kids' stuff, nor does it necessarily fade away at the age of twenty-one. It can linger well into prime-time adulthood or first flourish in the twenties, thirties, and even later. A recent British study cited in *Modern Medicine* found facial acne especially prevalent in men and women aged eighteen to sixty. Dermatologists estimate that from twenty to fifty percent of their acne patients are adults, who are just as susceptible as teenagers to its most severe forms, along with its devastating emotional effects.

Sometimes external circumstances are clearly to blame. One thirty-four-year-old woman who had enjoyed previously flawless skin was stricken with an explosive widespread condition after taking steroids for colitis; it is a known side effect of this medication. A dermatologist lanced and drained the pustular acne lesions and injected them with cortisone, but they returned soon after. Eventually her condition was brought under control by a combination of aggressive topical and oral treatments. Her facial scars can be minimized with a number of new techniques, but the psychological imprint will linger on.

"I never realized how acne or any skin disorder could

be so tied up with self-esteem and sexual attractiveness and how so many people tend to judge others by their appearance," she observes. "Having a bad case of acne is like being grossly overweight. In a similar way, people view it as the result of slovenliness or carelessness or being out of control, even though this is totally untrue. The state of my face affected the way I felt about myself and related to others. Although I realized my problem wasn't life-threatening, I would have traded it gladly for some internal disorder which nobody could see."

"While they're not as medically serious, most illnesses of the skin can be far more devastating to the psyche than systemic diseases," notes Dr. Michael Haberman, medical director of the department of psychiatry at Atlanta's West Paces Ferry Hospital, "Adult-onset diabetes can cost you your life, but it doesn't cause the kind of excruciating emotional trauma, the personal upheaval, that acne could. And the outbreak need not be severe. I know people who won't leave their houses out of embarrassment—a salesman who blew a very lucrative deal just because he had a big pimple on his nose. He felt humiliated and unworthy of success, a massive psychological reaction that dated back to what happened at his high-school party. He had had a classic, full-bloom case and was all but shunned by his classmates. So even one pimple years later was enough to trigger all those ugly memories for him."

Because of a number of competing, very powerful pressures, the adolescent is often thrown into a state of emotional turmoil. "He or she has to move toward independence, become an acceptable member of a peer group, cope with a changing body image—that's a tall order. Rejection or feelings of inadequacy at this time because of some real or imagined facial defect can be very damaging to a fragile, still-formative sense of self," Dr. Haberman adds.

As Dr. James Fulton reports in his book, *Farewell To Pimples,* a survey of over 1,000 suburban New York high school students found that the ones with acne complained most frequently of people staring at them, a feeling of isolation at parties and difficulty working with others. Unfortunately, a surprising number of those *without* acne believed that blemishes were largely the outward manifestation of "negative thoughts" and unclean habits—myths which could only reinforce the embarrassment and self-blame of their acne-troubled classmates! Similar results emerged from a Minnesota Multiphasic Personality Inventory test conducted at the University of Texas, where the students with acne were typically less confident, more withdrawn, depressed, and anxious about new social situations.

One twenty-seven-year-old patient who had battled a persistent case of acne since she was fourteen called it the most "unbelievably frustrating and demoralizing problem" of her life. "I was obsessed with my condition, literally a slave to my acne," she recalls. She would visit the mirror at least twenty-five times a day, leaving her desk at work for long stretches of time to wash her face "with a venegeance, while studying and agonizing over every pimple." Hers was no simple soap and water ritual. "I would scrub my face hard with very hot water until it got raw and red, even bleeding. I dreaded the routine because it was so uncomfortable, so time-consuming, but I thought by being aggressive I could just wipe away my acne. The harder I pushed, the worse it got."

The practice was so ingrained that she could not tolerate being away from the mirror more than a few hours—"away from sinks, washcloths, and all my other paraphernalia. Since I was vain to begin with, having such stubborn, noticeable acne was constant daily torture. I avoided looking people straight in the eye (I always stared at my shoes) and passed up invitations to parties. I really missed out on some good times socially because I was too absorbed with myself," she says regretfully. "Other people, especially my parents, would tell me it wasn't that terrible, that I was exaggerating and making a big fuss over nothing. My only answer to that was, It's very easy to downplay any problem that isn't yours. We may be our toughest critics, but no one else can even guess how awful acne feels unless they've experienced it themselves.''

Now, with the problem finally under control, she says, "My whole life and personality have changed because I can get through an entire day without looking at my face and crying.''

How Acne Begins

Although doctors do not know precisely why some people are plagued with acne flareups for years while others escape virtually unscathed, a closer look at the process can provide some clues.

From birth tiny oil-producing glands (sebaceous glands) lie buried beneath the skin almost everywhere except the palms and soles. The face, chest, and back, where acne most often occurs, harbor the highest concentration. As many as five thousand may be clustered on a given square inch of facial skin. During puberty the sudden surge of male hormones (called androgens) in both sexes that signals bodily change awakens the dormant glands. Though the resulting flow of oil does not automatically lead to acne, it sets the stage and no acne is possible without it.

However, some oily-skinned people have very little acne, while people with dry complexions can have a serious case, so the disease defies easy generalization. And while hormones play a leading role, usually no imbalance is involved. Only a small amount is needed to prod the oil glands, and it is impossible to distinguish the androgen levels of acne patients from those of clear-skinned types.

Think of an oil gland, or follicle, as shaped something like an upside-down cauliflower or mushroom, with a stem or duct attached to a bulbous base. The oil secreted at the base normally flows out through the duct to be deposited on the surface of the skin and washed away. Carried with it are the outer layers of dead cells lining the neck of the gland, which are regularly sloughed off as new ones form beneath. Acne occurs when this orderly traffic is interrupted. The layers of dead cells start to stick together, gradually forming a plug that blocks the oil's escape route. The bacteria normally present at the base of the gland thrive well in this dark, airless trap and begin to feed on the backed-up oil. These formerly friendly microbes turn destructive, unleashing an enzyme that breaks the oil down into so-called free fatty acids and other irritating by-products.

When the bulging cells, oil, and bacteria completely block the opening to the surface, the visible result is a tiny swollen bump called a closed comedo or whitehead. As the gland continues to expand, one of two things will happen. The plug may stretch the oil-gland walls apart near the top, forming the notorious blackhead (open comedo). Contrary to popular myth, the black part is caused by melanin, a dark skin pigment which deepens when exposed to air, *not* by dirt. Or the disease may progress to red, tender papules (pimples), pustules (white-capped pimples that have come to a head), and more deeply rooted nodules or cysts—all potentially scarring. These problem blemishes form when the debris within the glands exerts so much pressure that it breaks through the oil-gland walls, spilling into the dermis and inflaming the surrounding tissue. Scavenging white blood cells are summoned to stem the invasion, and the battle produces the unsightly surface results—redness, irritation, swelling, pus.

Since this whole process occurs about one-eighth of an inch below the skin, acne cannot simply be washed away. It is the oil that does not make it to the surface that causes all the trouble.

Recently people with chronically oily skin and lingering

acne have been found to harbor an especially active enzyme that converts testosterone, one of the androgens, into
a more potent form called dihydrotestosterone. This is the
factor directly responsible for releasing more oil. Scientists
speculate that acne may someday (soon) be controlled or
even prevented by counteracting the effects of dihydrotestosterone on the sebaceous glands. The challenge lies in
accomplishing this without tampering with the body's normal hormone makeup.

Genes are believed to play a stage-setting role, since
acne and its degree of severity often run in families (though
there are many exceptions). Heredity can help determine
the amount of oil your body produces, the kind of bacteria
nesting in your glands, the strength of your follicle walls,
and other factors linked to either your resistance or your
susceptibility. For example, identical twins who suffer
from acne get pimples at roughly the same time and to the
same degree. Some families seem to specialize in superficial whiteheads and blackheads; in others, the oil-gland
walls break down rapidly, the lesions are deep, and the
process is more inflammatory and cystic.

Occasionally the onset of acne in adulthood can signal
the presence of pituitary, adrenal, or ovarian tumors. The
condition will usually be accompanied by other signs of
excess androgen or erratic hormone activity: irregular menstrual periods, the growth of facial hair, deepening of the
voice, etc.

Other factors, if not direct causes, may aggravate an
already existing case of acne. For example, when assaulted
by anxiety and stress, the body signals the pituitary or
"master" gland to release more of its hormones to meet
the challenge. One of these, in turn, stimulates an area
called the adrenal cortex to pour more androgens into the
bloodstream. Since people vary in their tolerance to extra
androgens, not everyone under pressure will have an acne
flareup. But stress will put those who are susceptible at
higher risk.

Even more important, stress can lead to nervous, repetitive scratching and picking on or about the face, which can irritate pimples and drive them deeper into the skin. Dr. Samuel Frank of New York University has discovered that anxiety and anger increase the flow of oil in acne patients, while periods of tranquility tend to lower it substantially. The output of fatty acids has also been found to increase during stressful times.

Myths Versus Facts

Almost as plentiful and persistent as the causes of acne are the myths and misconceptions surrounding this still poorly understood condition. Some of these beliefs are groundless, while others need to be qualified with reliable fact.

Improper hygiene is a leading cause of acne. Nothing could be further from the truth. If anything, acne patients seem obsessed with washing and scrubbing, which ironically can make their condition worse if carried to excess. Cleansing lends a feeling of well-being and a sense that you are doing something active and positive about your condition. It removes only surface oils, which can block pore openings but are not the real culprits in acne.

Long hair can aggravate acne. The length of your hair is not related to the severity of the problem. However, hair should be washed regularly, since seborrhea often accompanies acne and scalp oils may drip onto the forehead. This can help block pores superficially and lead to itching and scratching, which will irritate already sensitive, broken-out skin.

Acne is more common among girls than boys. This only seems so. Girls and women are more likely to see a physician about their problem, since they are more conscious about their appearance than men. But acne occurs with the same frequency in both sexes. In fact, men are more often victims of severe cystic (conglobate) acne of the back and chest.

Acne is contagious. Though bacteria are implicated in acne, they are buried deep within the skin, and the condition is never catching.

Acne is the visible result of sexual frustration; a better life in bed will help clear up your skin. This myth has an especially stubborn history; not until 1949 was it scientifically disproved. But believers still abound. Alas, acne does not improve after sexual intercourse.

Masturbation makes acne worse. This is equally groundless. Self-stimulation will do nothing to make your condition either better or worse. Presumably guilt, particularly among adolescents, has kept this myth alive and well.

Eating certain foods can cause or aggravate acne. Recent testing has found diet largely blameless as a cause of acne. Even the traditionally "forbidden" foods, such as chocolate, colas, dairy products, and french fries, are no longer considered menaces to the face. Fats that have been eaten do not find their way to the skin directly, and fats within the oil glands do not resemble those circulating in your bloodstream, so, in theory even the greasiest foods are okay.

However, overindulging in iodide or androgen-rich foods, such as shellfish, seaweed, kelp, cabbage, artichokes, wheat germ, organ meats, and gluten bread, may trigger acnelike eruptions in certain sensitive people. But these reactions are relatively rare, and in general large amounts must be consumed before any damage is done.

A good dietary rule of thumb is this: If you notice a skin outbreak or extra oiliness after eating a particular food, cross it off your menu for a while. If your complexion clears, test the suspected food by eating it again. Take a normal portion and eat it on its own. If a similar flareup occurs, you may decide to avoid or cut down on that item in the future.

While a single food in isolation will rarely give rise to acne, the total diet may play more than a neutral role. A few intriguing studies have compared populations with markedly different eating patterns. For example, acne is far less prevalent in Kenya and Zambia than among young black Americans of comparable age. In South Africa, acne reportedly became a problem only after the Zulus migrated from village to town and had a new lifestyle to match. Consider the Eskimos, too, whose largely seafood diet became thoroughly "westernized" after World War II. Their new diet ran to sweets, red meats, soft drinks, and refined white flour. The result was civilized diseases— tooth decay and gum disease, obesity, acne, diabetes, atherosclerosis, and coronary artery disease—all formerly rare or nonexistent in this group. (Doctors believe that no specific foods are responsible; rather, it is the ratio of wholesome, unadulterated foods to fats and overly refined products that spells the difference.)

What is the connection between acne and diet, if any? One possible theory is this: A high intake of both fats and protein, typical affluent fare, has been linked with more rapid growth and earlier sexual development in boys and girls. A century ago, when most people had a more sparing, simple diet, menarche (first menstruation) usually came at sixteen or seventeen; today it comes at twelve and thirteen. Since it is the onrush of "maturing" hormones that sets the stage for acne, any diet that hastens their release is likely to promote rather than inhibit acne (if it has any influence at all). Some doctors speculate that acne in young, well-fed patients may result from excess oil being blocked by gland openings that are still too small and immature to handle the load.

The link between acne and your overall diet is not necessarily far-fetched. Scientists have already demonstrated the role of diet in a more serious disease, breast cancer. (This, too, tends to be far more prevalent in countries with high-fat, high-protein, and refined-food diets.)

Of course, until all the evidence is in, the best policy is still moderation. The recently established U. S. Dietary Goals are probably the most sensible and well-justified guidelines to date. These advise that you increase considerably your intake of fibrous complex carbohydrates (whole-grain breads and cereals, raw or minimally cooked fresh vegetables and fruits) and reduce both saturated and unsaturated fats, cholesterol, refined sugars, and sodium. No one knows whether the national acne rate would start to decline if everyone started to eat this way from birth. And no one can claim that making sweeping changes in your diet will clear up your acne any faster (though it probably can't hurt). But the prospect of greater vigor and better overall health make this way of eating certainly worth a try. (See Chapter 11 for a full discussion of diet and skin.)

Eating certain foods or taking special vitamins will make acne disappear. No one food or nutrient can ever clear up a sickness. The role of diet and supplements is to build and repair body tissues, sustain the processes vital to life, and help keep your system in good working order so that it has an adequate supply of energy and can keep illness at bay. Recent experiments have linked vitamin A with acne-clearing, but the effective oral doses are dangerously high and possibly lethal. Some interesting European studies suggest that modest amounts of zinc may play a beneficial role, but this is still untested theory. On the positive side, a sensible diet can only help strengthen your resistance to disease and allow you to cope better with an existing one.

The best supplement to every diet is a well-tempered lifestyle. Try to avoid or remove yourself from stressful situations. Get plenty of restful sleep. Learn to defuse tensions by relaxing at intervals throughout even the busiest working day; a total of ten or fifteen minutes is enough, and even a company president can spare this much time. Regular exercise will help release pent-up emotions and enliven skin tone by enhancing circulation.

If this lifestyle becomes a habit, it will be a strong ally when you mount an anti-acne offensive.

Acnelike Conditions

Rosacea

This chronic acnelike condition is most common among people of Celtic descent and generally affects adults, not adolescents. The characteristics are dilated capillaries, diffused redness, and firm, tender, deeply rooted acne-type papules. The pimply facial flushing and swelling is often symmetrically arranged, particularly around the nose, cheeks, and chin. W. C. Field's bulbous red nose was probably a "glowing example" of this disorder.

Although rosacea is quite common, its cause remains unclear. Mild gastrointestinal trouble and oral infections are sometimes linked with the condition. Treatment usually involves avoiding alcohol, coffee, tea, cola drinks, chocolate, and hot, spicy, or exotically seasoned foods, such as relishes, pickles, curried dishes, sharp sauces, sharp cheeses, mustard, chili, horseradish, all of which have a dilating effect on blood vessels. Also to be avoided are the sun and extremes of heat and cold—hot stoves, overheated interiors, icy winds. Oral infections should be eliminated, particularly those affecting the teeth and gums.

Rosacea is also often based on what might be called a chronically anxious frame of mind. Many patients suffer from "social anxiety," aware of the constant demands of conscience, duty, and obligation and feeling that they are not able to meet them. This creates a chronic depression that reduces the functions and efficiency of the whole system, especially the blood vessels of the face and stomach. Some pointers for a lasting recovery: Stop saying "you must" to yourself. Sidestep or resign from up to fifty percent of your committees, refuse drives, and be lazy—even irresponsible—often enough to give mind, conscience, and nerves a well-deserved rest. Be more satisfied with the day and the hour as they are. Stop striving for goals, feverishly trying to measure up to or surpass your expectations for yourself. (You might ask yourself, "A hundred years from now, what will this matter?") Always eat slowly and in peace, without worries on your mind, and avoid discussing household or business problems at meals.

Both systemic and local therapy can work wonders for rosacea. Oral tetracycline and topical benzoyl peroxide can reduce pustules and shrink distended vessels, while hydrocortisone creams and sulfur lotions can curb redness and related discomfort. A condition called rhinophyma, characteristic of severe rosacea, in which the nose becomes grotesquely enlarged with the acnelike growths and swollen vessels, can be treated with simple surgery, electrodesiccation and/or dermabrasion to sculpt it to its former size and shape.

Steroid Rosacea
This is a close cousin of the ordinary kind, but unlike the latter, never involves rhinophyma, and its lesions may

appear in unusual places, such as the eyelids and sides of the face.

Fluorinated topical steroid creams, which are often used to treat a local dermatitis or inflammation, have been singled out as the leading, if not only, cause in adults. Discontinuing this medication abruptly can result in a "rebound phenomenon" of the original condition which may last up to two weeks. A non-fluorinated steroid, such as a low-potency hydrocortisone cream, can be used to blunt the rebound effect. Anti-acne agents also help. After all steroids have been eliminated, oral tetracycline can pave the way for rapid clearing. (For children erythromycin or ampicillin should be prescribed instead.) Once therapy begins, steroid rosacea usually subsides slowly over several months.

Perioral Dermatitis

The presence of uniform tiny, itchy lesions around the mouth and chin (and occasionally the nose and eyes) may signal this other acne imitator, which occurs most commonly in younger women. The red or flesh-colored papules and pustules (the size of a pencil eraser) occur singly or in clusters. Alternatively the problem may erupt as persistent redness or swelling around the naso-labial fold (the groove between the nostrils and sides of the mouth). Perioral dermatitis is also readily confused with rosacea and seborrheic dermatitis (see page 46). Like the former, it may result from overusing fluorinated steroid medications, topical or systemic. Sunlight, cosmetics, heredity, and hormone activity are also possible culprits.

Since perioral dermatitis is often misdiagnosed, doctors may unwittingly make matters worse by prescribing an inappropriate regimen. (Drugstore acne remedies often aggravate this condition.) Systemic antibiotics usually work in three to eight weeks, though sometimes longer-term treatment with gradually lowered doses of the drugs is necessary. Cleansing with a mild soap and warm water, followed by a camphorated lotion, can help relieve discomfort.

Pyoderma Faciale
This is a misnamed and malevolent variant of acne conglobata (see page 65) which afflicts mostly women who are well past adolescence. The typically inflamed, very large nodules and excessive oiliness are confined to the face. Although no clear-cut cause has been uncovered, intense, prolonged anxiety or distress is a common theme in patients' histories. Victims frequently report such traumatic events as a death, loss of a job, and marital discord, leading many doctors to conclude that this disorder has a psychosomatic origin. For that reason, tranquilizers and psychotherapy may be prescribed along with the usual internal and topical treatments.

CHAPTER 4

Rx FOR MILD TO MODERATE ACNE

Whether your acne is simply an emotionally upsetting breakout or a full-blown, disfiguring dilemma, it should be dealt with promptly. The longer you delay, the greater your risk of being visibly scarred.

While some people are predestined by heredity to develop a severe condition, most can take active steps to avoid the external, environmental irritants and influences that can lead to the same result. Acne comes in many shapes and sizes, as the following categories suggest. All can be prevented if you are adequately forewarned.

Acne Cosmetica
If women outnumber men among adults with acne, it is because they are heavier users of cosmetics. Unfortunately some of the longest-lasting, best-concealing products contain derivatives of fatty acids and irritating oils that are potent acne stimulants. For example, many cosmetics include an expensive, penetrating ingredient that soaks deeply into pores, plugging up oil-gland openings. Called isoprophyl myristate, it is also the active component in Liquid Wrench, a product used by mechanics to loosen rusted bolts and nuts.

Lanolins (derived from sheepskin oil) and detergents, such as sodium laurel sulfate, hexadecyl alcohol, hexylene glycol, and polyethylene glycol, are also irritants if used for prolonged periods. When deposited on the sensitive ears of rabbits, they give rise to acne-type eruptions fairly quickly. In fact, the rabbit ear experiment has been used to test the acne-producing potential of a wide variety of agents, including foundations, cleansing and cold creams, moisturizers, suntan oils, hand lotions, astringents, blushers, and hair pomades. As well as physically blocking pores and preventing the escape of sebum, some makeups contain ingredients that instigate acne by affecting the cells lining the oil glands. A grade, or comedogenic assay number, from 0 to 2 means that a cosmetic has few or no acne-causing properties, while a number from 3 to 5 denotes a significant to severe potential. Many products have been rated this way. Before buying a facial formula, ask at the cosmetics counter about its acne potential.

Ironically many women use heavy cosmetics and vanishing creams to conceal their acne, only to find that these trigger still more outbreaks, leading to a vicious cycle. Frequently, even after a product is discontinued, it takes several months for the blemishes to disappear.

What can you do, short of spending your life barefaced—which is highly unlikely and not much fun? Since not all cosmetics will affect you adversely, experiment until you find the one that is right for you. Water-based and oil-free foundations are your safest bets. You can usually recognize the former as liquids that separate when not in use and have to be shaken. Because oil-free (alcohol-based) makeups contain emulsifiers (which hold the ingredients together), they are less likely to cake or turn pasty than the water-based kinds. However, the emulsifiers that make them more cosmetically elegant aggravate existing acne in certain people. The answer is to try an oil-free foundation if you find it more appealing, but study your face closely and switch brands if one product seems to provoke an outbreak. Generally, makeups containing pigments, water, glycerin, alcohol, and propylene glycol are best for acne-prone skin.

Consult this list of troublemaking ingredients before reading your next cosmetic label.

> isopropyl isostearate
> butyl stearate
> myristyl myristate
> isopropyl palmitate
> isocetyl stearate
> decyl oleate
> isostearyl neopentanoate
> octyl stearate
> octyl palmitate
> isopropyl lanolate
> acetol acetulan
> amberate P
> crude coal tar
> lanosterin
> langogene
> sterolan
> PG 2 myristyl propionate
> acetylated lanolin
> ethyloxylated lanolin
> D & C red dyes (common in blushers)

The terms "dermatologist-tested," "hypoallergenic," and "medicated" can all be falsely reassuring, since the preparation to which they refer may contain one or more of the forbidden agents mentioned above. And expensive, highly elegant cosmetics may be more comedogenic than cruder, cheaper ones. You can do your own testing of cosmetics by smearing a portion onto a piece of dull-finish cotton bond paper or a brown paper bag and examining it under light the following day. Avoid the product if the sample shows streaks of oil.

One final point on acne and cosmetics. Often women past thirty assume that flaking means dryness, but excessively oily skin can peel and scale as well (a condition called seborrheic dermatitis). For this reason avoid radical dry-skin regimens that call for heavy moisturizing creams. Remember, skin is most often a combination of types, so any extreme approach—over-lubricating or over-drying— may lead to either an aggravated case of acne or excessive irritation.

Acne Mechanica

Continual irritation, pressure, and friction caused by leaning hands against the face, holding musical instruments, wearing tight sweatbands, football padding, headgear, backpacks or shoulder straps, even casts and bandages, can aggravate an existing case of acne and heighten the risk of scarring. It can also dislodge noninflammatory lesions or microcomedones—tiny "time bombs" waiting to erupt beneath the surface—and result in new outbreaks. One theory is that excessive pressure concentrates moisture on the skin surfaces, which causes cells in the outer layers to swell. This reduces the size of pore openings and makes it harder for oils to exit. Vigorous brushing and combing of hair is another mechanical acne stimulus, since it can rupture microscopic glands and release scalp oils onto the face.

Be alert to the unconscious habits and mannerisms that aggravate acne. For example, avoid resting your head in your hands while studying, reading, or watching television. It is no coincidence that right-handed people often have more blemishes on the right side of their face. Some people repeatedly rub or knead a particular spot, especially when under stress, and usually are surprised when this automatic activity is brought to their attention. But just becoming aware of certain gestures or behaviors is often enough to put an end to them.

One possible clue to the cause of acne mechanica is lesions that are distributed in an unusual or telltale pattern— for example, a swath of pimples across the forehead or symmetrical outbreaks over both shoulders.

A nurse developed acne mechanica as a result of wearing tight surgical masks whenever she assisted during operations. Acutely embarrassed by her acne, she took to wearing her mask more often than necessary so that no one would notice it—a habit that only perpetuated her condition.

Fast Food Acne

This condition is common among people who work near the cooking area in fast-food chains and are continually exposed to flying grease. Machine oils and cutting greases used by auto machanics, along with coal tar dyes, dandruff shampoos, and insecticides, are also powerful acne catalysts.

Chemical Acne

Kelp, spinach, seaweed, and shellfish, all of which contain iodides and fluorides, can make acne worse if eaten in large amounts. The same is true of medicines that contain bromides (some asthma and cold remedies), salicylates (such as aspirin), barbiturates or tranquilizers.

Large doses of estrogens will shut down the oil glands, which is why many pregnant women and women on high-dose hormone contraceptives watch their acne disappear. However, the newer, safer, low-estrogen pills also contain progesterone, which has a sebum-stimulating effect on the body. And withdrawal from either kind of pill may cause a sudden flareup due to a rebound reaction as the body adjusts to new hormone levels.

Steroid Acne

Sustained internal corticosteroid therapy can cause this variant of chemical acne. It is marked by an all-over-the-body reaction (including places where ordinary acne almost never appears), usually in the form of tiny pustules. Sometimes application of potent corticosteroid creams to the face and body can have a similar effect.

Vitamin Acne

Watch out for preparations containing bromides or iodides. Ask your pharmacist or physician for guidance if labels are unclear. A highly inflammatory form of acne is a not uncommon risk for anemic women who require frequent injections of vitamin B_{12}. B_{12} may contain traces of iodine that remain in commercial preparations after the process used to extract the vitamin. The acne clears spontaneously within eight to ten days of the therapy being discontinued.

Tropical Acne

Intense heat and humidity often lead to excessive sweating; the increased moisture combined with surface oils can irritate existing lesions and spur new outbreaks. Also, sebum spreads more rapidly over a wet surface.

In addition, the term "tropical acne" is used for a ravaging eruptive condition that is even more painfully disfiguring than acne conglobata. The victims are invariably young men, usually soldiers stationed in the tropics for extended periods of time. They sweat profusely while clothed and have to endure friction or pressure from tight, wet clothing. Even the most powerful combination of medications has no impact. The only remedy is to leave the hot, humid environment immediately.

Acne Mallorca

A kind of acne actually induced by sunbathing. While many dermatologists advise their patients to soak up sunlight, its effects can be contradictory. It evens out skin color (thereby camouflaging pimples), dries up surface oils, and causes mild peeling. But it may also lead to a crop of new comedones several weeks after exposure. In fact, September and October are often a dermatologist's busiest months. Acne kept in temporary check by summer sun may erupt even more explosively later on. No one is sure why, but some dermatologists believe that too much tanning thickens skin, creating a layer of hard-to-slough cells that clog pores and follicles, thus setting up a perfect environment for comedones.

Solar blackheads frequently show up on older adult white skin after excessive sun exposure, especially around the eyes and cheeks. Sometimes these enlarge enough to look like cysts on a background of yellowish, thickened, and loose-hanging skin, a condition known as morbus Favre-Racouchot (solar damage to the elastic tissue of the dermis). In this case, hair follicles and sebaceous glands open and sizable blackhead-like lesions are formed as dead skin cells and pigment are trapped inside.

The solution is to bask in moderate doses of sunshine with a non-comedogenic sunscreen, such as Sunguard, Pre-Sun, Eclipse, Sundown, Panabol, or Paragel, which will block out the most skin-damaging rays while your condition improves.

Working Women's Acne

The majority of women now work outside the home and more are assuming positions of executive responsibility. Acne (usually an aggravated case of existing oiliness) is one often overlooked consequence. Driven, Type A women and men, chronically demanding and impatient, and stubbornly obsessive about their jobs, may allow themselves few creative and emotional outlets and as a result have frequent flareups of acne. It is as if their skin were erupting from all their pent-up problems and pressures.

Detergent Acne

Too frequent or vigorous scrubbing with detergents and abrasive soaps can irritate already broken-out skin. Do not confuse thorough cleansing with harsh cleansing. And never use rough washcloths, loofahs, or oatmeal grains on an acne-studded face. Sometimes people with the mildest cases will scrub the hardest, probably because they believe a little extra effort will eliminate the problem together.

The benefits of washing are largely psychological. The cooling and tingling sensations refresh, washing removes the shine that magnifies defects, and the ritual itself convinces the acne sufferer that he or she is taking a positive step.

Acne Excoriée des Jeunes Filles

This is a self-inflicted problem (meaning literally "excoriated acne of young girls"), which usually begins in adolescence. An isolated pimple or cluster may be singled out for vigorous scratching, squeezing, and picking in order to make it disappear. Or else a patient may simply gouge out imaginary pimples. The frequent result is deep and irregular linear scars.

Acne excoriée can occur in both sexes at almost every age, but adolescent females are most susceptible. More than a simple unconscious tic or mannerism, it often stems from deep-seated anxieties, a lack of confidence and self-esteem, or even sexual hangups. Marring a basically unblemished face is one way to withdraw socially, to reinforce a flawed self-image, or to account for lack of popularity with the opposite sex. It can also be a way of freeing oneself from guilt. Such people usually benefit more from intensive emotional counseling and support than conventional treatment.

Pomade Acne

This is a variation of acne cosmetica and is caused by expensive hair formulas with high-grade ingredients. It takes the form of a densely crowded mass of whiteheads, mainly on forehead and temples. The best approach is to see a dermatologist and switch to much simpler grooming aids. Cream rinses and conditioners are quite as effective as greases and oils. Apply them sparingly to the ends of the hairs, not to the scalp.

If caught early enough, about one half of all acne cases, regardless of their origin, can be controlled by over-the-counter treatments. Conscientious home care (and prompt medical attention when necessary) can spell the difference betewen proliferating lesions that result in scars and normal skin with only an occasional flareup.

Cleansing Guidelines

Since acne is not caused by dirt, overzealous washing does not clear the skin. The oils, dead cells, and bacterial by-products do their mischief about two millimeters below the surface, beyond the reach of even the strongest soap. However, oils on the skin can inhibit healing by blocking the flow of sebum. To remove them, wash gently with a mild soap. A heavy, abrasive touch will only inflame already sensitive skin and rupture follicle walls, releasing new comedones. Use the tips of your fingers to lather your face, and rinse thoroughly with tepid water. Pat or blot dry with a smooth-surfaced cloth or tissue; do not rub.

One formerly fanatical scrubber, who had managed to redden and blister her already acne-ravaged face, noticed a dramatic change in texture soon after she adopted a gentler approach. "Once I started lathering lightly, my skin began to feel softer, more tender—less leathery and coarse," she reports. "A more 'civilized' way of cleansing was an important part of the cure!"

Remember your skin type and wash, as described in Chapter 2. Only light, grease-free moisturizers and astringents are acceptable for faces with acne, and the old standbys are still the best. Urea- or glycerin-based moisturizers, alcohol or witch hazel formulas for astringents. Astringents should be diluted with water if your face is especially flaky, dry, or sensitive. (While mild astringents give local, bracing relief by clearing surface oil and stimulating circulation, so-called pore-minimizers can sometimes aggravate acne by causing a slight local swelling. This temporarily decreases pore openings and so partially blocks the escaping sebum.)

Since acne is often a companion to seborrhea, wash your hair at least every other day with a mild, oil-controlling (alkaline) shampoo and style it away from your face, if possible. Change your pillowcase frequently, since natural oils from both scalp and face may accumulate there.

Caution: Never pick or squeeze pimples or attempt to remove them yourself with a store-bought comedone extractor. This is a tricky, delicate procedure, which should be performed by professional hands only.

Most people do their compulsive picking on a wet, soapy face while looking in the bathroom mirror. To avoid the temptation, pat your face dry immediately after washing and do not linger to examine yourself. Apply a water-based or oil-free makeup to conceal pimples from both yourself and others.

To men: When shaving, you may be tempted to nick one or two small pimples, since only minimal bleeding will result. But you can't eradicate acne by removing the tip; it's like breaking off a weed instead of digging up the roots. And you will only risk more serious inflammation and permanent scarring. Before shaving, wet the skin thoroughly to soften follicles, then apply cream or mild soap.

To root out the "one big pimple," particularly the white-capped variety or pustule that crops up almost diabolically before an all-important date or social gathering, pour boiling water into a bowl or sink and bend your face over it to catch the steam. After the water has cooled slightly, add 1 teaspoon of salt for every pint of water; dab the affected area 10 to 15 times with a clean washcloth dipped in the salt water. Then apply cotton soaked in alcohol or witch hazel (or the juice of a lemon or tomato if your medicine chest is empty). Repeat as necessary. Repeated warm water soaks followed by drying will increase blood flow, help reduce inflammation, and promote the draining of pustules.

A large, angry-red pimple that is not yet on the verge of ripening can be treated in a dermatologist's office with an injection of a dilute corticosteroid. Since it is delivered with a small-gauge needle, most patients hardly feel it; generally the lesion will shrink in one to two days. The benefit of such acne surgery is that it helps reduce some of the most visible blemishes, eliminating the temptation to pick and thus indirectly preventing scarring.

Beyond Soap: Special Acne Cleansers

Many people with acne feel obligated to use something more powerful and "medicinal" than ordinary soap. Are the array of special cleansers lining pharmacists' shelves worth the extra investment?

A recent survey of over-the-counter products by the Food and Drug Administration (with results published in *Consumer Reports*) found the majority of medicated anti-acne soaps, scrubs, and lotions completely ineffective.

While many products claim to be "deep-pore" cleansers, pores are merely surface openings; acne originates far below them. No soap can penetrate to the skin's troubled lower layers, so the term is misleading and meaningless. Other cleansers boast of antibacterial power. While this may sound medically persuasive, the irritating microbes in acne do most of their damage in the absence of oxygen; they operate deep within the follicle walls, not on the surface of the skin.

The popular abrasive scrubs contain particles of polyethylene or aluminum for stripping away outer cells. But like rough-textured pads and washcloths, these may do more harm than good by scouring already sensitive skin. Sulfur and benzoyl peroxide are effective topical ingredients when allowed to penetrate the skin. But in soaps and cleansers they have little value, since they are so quickly washed away. Most of the antiseptic cleansers and lotions contain alcohol, which will soak up outer oils and dead skin cells along with local bacteria. But none of this directly combats acne, and ordinary soaps do a far better job of surface cleansing.

If your acne is confined to scattered blackheads or papules and shows no signs of severe inflammation, a number of store-bought formulas will help keep it under control. According to the Food and Drug Administration advisory panel, only three of twenty-eight active ingredients (sorted out from eighty-six chemicals used today) were judged safe and effective in home treatment of acne: sulfur, the combination sulfur-resorcinol, and benzoyl peroxide. Although the panel was divided on the issue, add salicylic acid to the list, since it is a potent peeling and drying agent with a worthy track record.

Sulfur, resorcinol, salicylic acid
These are long-standing remedies, used either alone or in combination. Such products' main value lies in drying out and layering away existing pimples, often dramatically reducing the time it takes for them to heal. Most are also tinted a flesh color for maximum camouflage.

Note: None of these products should ever be applied around the eyelids, under the chin, or on the neck, where skin is most delicate and easily irritated. Those with black and deep-toned skin should shy away from products containing sulfur and resorcinol, since both can cause pigment changes. Be careful to use only 2 percent strength formulas of salicylic acid. Preparations designed for warts and callouses generally contain much more. Do not use these products for acne; they can severely irritate, even ulcerate, facial skin.

Benzoyl Peroxide

This is the most promising drugstore solution so far (also available by prescription). Formulated in varying strengths, from 2.5 percent to 10 percent, it has the power to penetrate deeply into the troubled oil glands. There it releases oxygen, thereby killing off the oxygen-shy bacteria and curbing the destructive free fatty acids they produce. It also helps prevent new pimples from forming by peeling away upper skin layers. Some benzoyl products include special oil-absorbing agents for more dramatic results. To minimize irritation, adults with dry, sensitive skin should try the lower strengths first, as should people with fair skin, freckles, and red hair.

Be careful to note the expiration date on the package, since benzoyl peroxide is volatile and loses its potency very readily when exposed to air or left on the shelf too long. The strength of a 10 percent product might have diminished dramatically by the time you buy it. Also, avoid cream-based versions, since these may only aggravate acne by blocking pores. The most stable, drying, and best-penetrating vehicle is the gel form. Currently available are such over-the-counter benzoyl peroxide preparations as Oxy-5 and Oxy-10, Topex, and Dry & Clear, or Acnomex or Clearasil, Fostex BPO and Clear By Design.

Since benzoyl peroxide has a preventive effect, make

sure to apply the product even where no pimples are visible. Remember, hundreds of microcomedones may be hidden from view beneath the skin, waiting to explode. So the best approach is to cover every surface area where acne might develop, and that means the entire face, from hairline to jaw, along with the upper chest and back.

Beware of too much burning and peeling; prolonged discomfort can aggravate your case and discourage you from following through. However, some irritation, tightness, and dryness is a sign that the product is doing its work. The idea is to expose and toughen the skin in gradual stages, to build up tolerance slowly. Start with a thin film; at the beginning, three or four hours may be all you can tolerate before you have to wash the product off. After a week or ten days, you might apply it twice or three times a day. If the skin becomes too raw or inflamed, discontinue the treatment for a day or two and then use less frequently until you harden the skin sufficiently. Avoid sensitive areas, such as the upper lip, corners of the mouth, nasal folds, and skin near the eyes and earlobes. Always apply at least thirty minutes after washing, since moisture intensifies irritation. Expect to wait at least three or four weeks before noting any visible improvement.

Above all, be a conscientious, label-reading consumer. Follow all package instructions and discard any medication that causes undue irritation after more than a week of use. While some soreness is inevitable, persistent, painful inflammation signals skin in distress, not rapid healing. Also, avoid venturing into the sun without a sunscreen or foundation makeup that lists a sun-protection agent as one of the ingredients. Drying and peeling products strip away your protective outer layers of skin, leaving you more vulnerable than ever to dangerous ultraviolet radiation.

Some acne patients mistakenly believe they are allergic to benzoyl peroxide. But the problem might be that they use the product just before going to bed; some of it gets smeared on their pillow and touches their eyelids or other sensitive areas. The solution is to apply the benzoyl peroxide earlier in the evening and to change pillowcases frequently.

Keep in mind that one complexion may react differently from another to a given preparation. Remember, pigment loss and splotchiness are potential problems among the black, oriental, and tawny-skinned. If discoloration persists, see a dermatologist.

Facial Salons

Should you visit a facial salon to clear your acne? The advertised promises are undeniably tempting. Most frequently touted are special "deep-cleansing masks" and sweat-inducing "facial saunas." A facial sauna is a steamy vapor released by an electrical unit that heats water; the word "sauna" is misleading, since the heat applied is moist, not dry. Moisture cannot penetrate below a few superficial layers of skin and perspiration does not flush out impurities from skin; it may even make acne worse.

To put it simply, pampering yourself with a sauna treatment may relax and uplift you psychologically, but it is no substitute for soap and water, nor will it accelerate healing. And, despite claims, there's no evidence that gently stimulated, sauna-treated skin will absorb medications more readily or effectively than usual.

As for benefits, a mask causes superficial peeling, which may improve your acne slightly; it can also help curb surface oils and be a pleasantly invigorating way to supplement everyday cleansing. However, patients who use a mask without consulting a doctor first may risk making their skin overly sensitive to the medications he is prescribing. (For descriptions of different masks, see Chapter 10.)

CHAPTER 5

Rx FOR MODERATE TO SEVERE ACNE

If you are battling more than scattered pimples or blackheads around forehead or chin, if outbreaks are tender and inflamed or still spreading after months of home treatment, consider taking your case to a good dermatologist, preferably someone experienced in a wide range of acne problems. When started early enough, medical care can check a potentially serious condition before it gets worse and prevent the pits and pockmarks that inflammatory acne so often leaves behind.

Even when enlisting professional help, remember that just as no single factor alone accounts for acne, no one-shot strategy can guarantee success. Only a custom-tailored treatment that considers your personal acne history, skin type, family background, lifestyle, habits, chronic pressures at work or school, among other details, will ensure the best results. To have any lasting impact, treatment may also demand considerable time and perseverance, and also teamwork on the part of you and your doctor. Unfortunately, by failing to emphasize this point, too many physicians lose their patients before therapy has had a chance to work.

For everyone a multifaceted approach to acne is the surest route to rapid healing. This involves reducing the outflow of sebum within the glands, rooting out the bacteria, preventing dead skin cells from clumping together, and keeping the surface clear of oils that can block escaping sebum. To accomplish all this, the doctor's arsenal includes both oral and topical antibiotics, more powerful benzoyl peroxides, acne surgery, and a relatively new weapon, Retin A (vitamin A acid or tretinoin), applied externally. Both the oral and highly effective topical medications at the doctor's disposal can treat existing acne and prevent new lesions from forming.

Antibiotics

The well-known tetracycline family of antibiotics kills the bacteria nesting within the follicles whose enzymes break down the oil into fatty acids, the basic fuel for the acne process. These drugs, prescribed for over thirty years, are among the safest and best tested around.

If your case calls for tetracycline, you will usually be started on a dosage of about 250 milligrams to be taken two to four times daily. Since it is best absorbed on an empty stomach, the drug should be taken between meals, at least one hour before or two hours after a meal. Never swallow tetracyclines with milk or any other dairy food, iron supplements, or antacids. All these substances bind themselves to the medication, cancelling its effects. Also, never take the drug with other antibiotics, since the combination can severely upset your normal intestinal flora (the natural, beneficial bacteria residing there). If you are simultaneously undergoing treatment for another condition, make sure you tell both doctors what medications and dosages you are taking. Among the possible complications for tetracycline—which usually disappear when the dosage is reduced—are abdominal cramps, frequent soft stools or diarrhea, greater sensitivity to sunlight, and quite commonly excessive vaginal discharge triggered by an increased growth of monilia, a normal vaginal yeast.

Tetracyclines should be avoided outright by people with liver or kidney disease and also by pregnant women, for they may cause skeletal problems in the fetus and tooth discoloration.

It is a good idea to have periodic blood checks if you must take large doses for an extended period of time.

Oral antibiotics do not work as quickly against acne as they do against sore throats and earaches. It may take three to six weeks before your face shows any improvement. Eventually you will have fewer pimples and reduced inflammation. Occasionally, acne bacteria develop a resistance to tetracycline, which explains why some people fail to respond to it. In such cases, minocycline, a more powerful, longer-lasting (and more expensive) antibiotic is often an excellent alternative. An advantage of minocycline therapy is that it is not necessary to forgo milk and milk products, since these do not interfere with the drug's absorption from the intestine. However, it is far more expensive than tetracycline, four times the cost or more, depending on the dosage.

Acne Surgery

If you have a faceful of comedones (blackheads and whiteheads), your doctor may remove a few of the more obvious ones manually). His instrument is a slender metal extractor with a small loop attached to one end. Whiteheads or closed comedones are generally first opened with a fine needle before being lifted out. Some swelling may result, which normally subsides in one or two days. The resulting boost is probably more psychological than aesthetic. The slight but immediate visible improvement makes you feel better about your looks and your prognosis, which encourages you to continue the rest of the treatment. The procedure is also performed as a rescue measure to erase an unsightly pimple or two that have erupted before a big social event.

Be aware that this kind of surgery requires delicate, well-trained hands. Even experienced doctors can inflict scars by applying too much pressure or lifting out lesions with a sloppy technique. That is why extractions should be limited and reserved for emergencies only. Never do it yourself; you risk permanent pitting and scarring.

Acne surgery also involves lancing and draining large cysts, injecting them with minute amounts of corticosteroids, or both, to reduce their size. Results can be dramatic, with swelling markedly diminished often within twelve hours.

Sometimes pimples are sprayed with liquid nitrogen, Freon, or dry ice to hasten peeling, a procedure known as cryotherapy or cryosurgery. A local frostbite results which kills upper-layer cells and accelerates the normal shedding process. The treatment also minimizes scarring and camouflages lesions by reducing redness.

Cans of Freon can be stored at home and used by a reliable patient after thorough instructions and practice sessions (including videotapes and a demonstration) have been given in the doctor's office. Ask your doctor about this possibility. For best results hold the can about 5 inches from the acne-afflicted skin and spray for about 2 seconds on the face and 3 or 4 seconds on the chest, shoulders, and back. (You will probably get better results if you have someone else do the spraying for you.)

Vitamin A Acid

While vitamin A has long been recognized for its anti-acne properties, it can be toxic if taken in massive doses over an extended period of time, damaging eyes, liver, bones, gonads, and thyroid. Recently scientists pulled the vitamin apart to isolate its skin-healing benefits from its dangerous side effects and came up with two highly promising derivatives: topical vitamin A acid and a still-experimental oral drug called 13-cis-retinoic acid. The former, marketed as Retin-A, is a powerful face-peeler that seeps into the pores and essentially loosens the cells of the epidermis and hair follicle-oil gland (pilosebaceous) unit, where the acne process originates. It does this by reducing the cells' tendency to stick together and causing them to be shed more rapidly. The effect is to break apart existing lesions and prevent the formation of new ones.

Like benzoyl peroxide, vitamin A acid is an aggressive irritant the benefits of which are not readily noticeable. In fact, during the first few weeks of therapy, the rapidly drying, peeling, itching pimples may actually appear worse than ever. The skin will be rough, red, and flaky, and a decidedly unattractive crop of lesions will bloom quite prolifically for a while. The comedones and pimples are coming to a head at an accelerated rate, "exploding" out of their hidden chambers below. This initial outburst, which can last up to about four weeks, is followed by rapid healing, and a maintenance dose (two to three times weekly) may be sufficient to suppress future flareups.

Fast-Track Therapy

For many patients a combination of topical vitamin A and benzoyl peroxide gel is the most potent anti-acne formula around. The latter toughens the skin and reduces the irritating effects of the acid, while the vitamin A, in turn, enhances the antibacterial activity of the benzoyl peroxide. (Benzoyl is generally applied in the morning to prime the face, and vitamin A in the evening or on alternating nights.) Make sure you are secure enough to withstand the possibly unsightly immediate results before you submit to this fast-track, two-drug onslaught. Oil-free or water-based cosmetics can help camouflage the redness and chapping in the meantime. If you are seeing a dermatologist, ask for the latest list of approved non-comedogenic agents.

Also, be certain your doctor will be available to answer questions about your appearance and progress during this aggressive course of treatment. Some doctors, short on time or patience or with a high-volume practice, hesitate to prescribe new types of medication that require continual communication and feedback in order to succeed. Others do prescribe them, but fail to provide enough guidance and follow-through advice. Insist on both; they are indispensable to the "cure." And keep in mind that no two people react precisely alike to the same concentration or proportion of ingredients. Both vitamin A and benzoyl peroxide are available in several different strengths and bases, so treatment can be carefully suited to your needs. If a variety of one or the other is not effective or too harsh for you, tell your doctor promptly.

Another key to making this regimen work is preventing the skin from drying out, especially during cold, windy weather and low-humidity days. One interesting study has found that too much surface dryness apparently inhibits, rather than enhances, acne clearing. For maximum comfort, use an oil-free moisturizing cleanser such as Cetaphil (without water) and protect the face with an emollient, preferably right before showering, shampooing, or strenuous exercising. As with benzoyl, never apply vitamin A acid immediately after washing, since moisture only increases burning and irritation. Wait at least thirty minutes.

Also, avoid direct exposure to sunlight, since the vitamin A has caused you to shed a protective layer of skin along with the plugged-up oil glands. During treatment always use a protective sunscreen before venturing outdoors (a greaseless gel is best). Stay away from topical lotions containing alcohol, such as astringents and aftershaves, for these may only further inflame the thinned-out, sensitive skin. And try not to dab Retin-A around your eyes, in the folds of skin at the edges of your nose and ears, under your chin, or near the corners of your mouth. Since the skin tends to dry more easily in winter, you may need to apply the medication less frequently or use a milder product in colder weather.

Topical Antibiotics

In the past, topical antibiotics for acne proved disappointing, because the skin is just as capable of screening out antibacterial agents as harmful microbes. But the newest formulas can penetrate better and with far more promising results. In fact, when compared for effectiveness, topical and oral varieties have scored similar gains, according to some observers.

A recent survey of over five hundred dermatologists showed clindamycin to be the most widely used and best regarded topical around. And a controlled study found it just as potent as a low-dose oral tetracycline (500 mgs. a day) for inflammatory acne. Apart from minor stinging and burning and some temporary splotchiness, few side effects have been reported.

New Breakthrough for Cystic Acne

The most raging, explosive form of the disease is acne conglobata, which is characterized by large, often painful cysts and lingering inflammation. For some 350,000 victims it is an undeniably ugly, devastating disorder that affects men more frequently than women; all the victims have markedly oily skin and oversized sebaceous glands. Unfortunately this punishing variety does not necessarily begin or end with adolescence. It may persist uncontrollably well into the thirties and beyond. Conglobate acne generally takes root most violently on the back and chest, the lower part of the face, and the neck. Its legacy of huge, irregular scars is eloquent evidence of its tendency to invade large areas of skin. In some cases the disorder may signal a more serious, systemic illness, such as osteomyelitis, or an underlying defect in the immune system. A persistent multiple regimen of antibiotics, topical medications, and corticosteroid injections, along with incisions and drainage, can often yield dramatic results.

But occasionally severe cystic acne remains resistant to even the most aggressive methods. In such special cases, the new oral extract, 13-cis-retinoic acid, called Accutane, may be the solution. Taken in pill form, it has already proven powerfully effective for a majority of trial subjects. In one study, for example, it completely banished the cystic acne lesions of 13 out of 14 people and was 90 percent successful in the last case. Everyone's skin remained clear for at least five years—long after the drug had been discontinued! This long-term effect in the absence of medication was even more remarkable than the initial results. Since this early trial, Accutane has been given to more than 500 patients, all of whom have shown either marked improvement or complete recovery—most dramatically on the face—and lasting remissions in the absence of the drug.

The compound works—often within weeks or months—by curbing the activity of the sebaceous glands and thereby reducing the flow of oil. It can reportedly lower sebum production by as much as 80 percent (compared with reductions of about 30 percent for estrogen). Accutane also decreases the number of bacteria (called P. acnes) on the skin surface. Recently approved by the FDA, oral retinoic acid can at least be a very potent adjunct in the treatment of severe cystic acne, if not an outright "cure." However, it should only be considered a last-resort approach since the catalogue of possible side effects is quite extensive, ranging from mild to serious: cracking and inflammation of the lips, dryness of mucous membranes, frequent nose bleeds, conjunctivitis, joint pain, hair thinning, rashes, skin peeling, especially on palms and soles, general gastrointestinal complaints, fatigue, headache, increased susceptibility to sunburn and hypertriglyceridemia (elevated blood levels of fats called triglycerides, a potential risk factor in heart disease).

The knockout drug is also teratogenic—capable of causing birth defects—so women of childbearing age beware! Either the near-absolute protection provided by the Pill or total abstinence(!) is advised if you're considering Accutane. And, because no one knows whether the drug is excreted in human milk, it should *not* be given to nursing mothers. (Women should remain on contraceptives at least one month after treatment is discontinued.)

Patients on Accutane should be carefully monitored with a series of blood tests (often repeated several times during the first month of treatment) to check for a possible rise in triglycerides, among other factors. Add this costly procedure to the already steep price for a typical four-month course of treatment, plus the cost of required doctor visits and other expensive continuing therapy—topical lotions, oral antibiotics, and intralesional steroid injections—and you have a rather hefty medical investment.

Some people benefit from a second or even third four-month regimen, but an eight week, drug-free interval should be allowed between treatment periods to evaluate the effects of the drug. Remember, some faces may look decidedly worse during the early stages of therapy, before the skin shows any signs of clearing. Accutane may also lower your skin's tolerance to certain topical agents, making them feel too harsh and drying, and possibly calling for a switch to milder formulas.

Unfortunately, we are almost certain that this drug will be misused because of all the recent media emphasis on its role as an acne cure-all. We repeat: Accutane is a drastic, last-resort treatment intended only for the most severe and resistant acne conditions—not the ordinary kind! And it must never be borrowed from or passed on to relatives and friends—an all-too-common temptation among patients unaware of its powerful and potentially hazardous effects.

Fortunately, while not uncommon, any adverse reactions to the drug are chiefly dose-related and usually disappear when the therapy is either reduced or discontinued.

Another treatment that has worked in resistant cases is combining tetracycline with an anti-leprosy drug called Dapsone. Dapsone enables a doctor to use lower doses of the antibiotic than would normally be necessary when it is used on its own to treat a raging form of acne. Since it is undesirable to take very high doses of any antibiotic for prolonged periods, the Dapsone-tetracycline combination provides a safer alternative. Before beginning Dapsone, laboratory tests are essential, as well as close monitoring by a physician.

Ultraviolet Light

Some dermatologists, convinced of the sun's healing effect on acne, treat their patients with sunlamps. But the value of ultraviolet light has recently been debated. While it promotes mild peeling and drying, its chief benefit is to darken skin, merely making pimples less noticeable. The problem lies in deciding how much is beneficial; an excess can age the skin prematurely and make it more susceptible to cancer.

If UV therapy is used, exposure should be very carefully timed and kept strictly to a minimum. One acne patient has reported that her doctor kept her under a sunlamp and then proceeded to forget about her; there was no automatic timer and no nurse or assistant on hand to supervise. Make sure this does not happen to you.

Hormone Therapy

Progesterone is a female hormone with an androgen-like or oil-stimulating effect. For this reason some doctors prescribe high estrogen/low progesterone oral contraceptives for women patients with severe cystic acne that is resistant to other forms of therapy. (Estrogen's effects are too "feminizing" to allow its use on men.)

The obvious drawback to this approach are the risks associated with the birth control pill, including greater susceptibility to blood clots and other circulatory disorders, endometrial cancer and gall bladder disease, nausea and weight gain. Make sure your acne is stubborn enough to warrant such a drastic therapy and that you are closely monitored and kept on the treatment for a limited period (approximately six months). A significant number of women are not helped by the Pill, and there is no way of telling beforehand who will and who won't respond. Sometimes results are not visible for at least four or five months. In fact, your face may look worse initially.

If you are already on the Pill and are trying to control

your acne, discuss your skin problem with your gynecologist, since some high-progesterone varieties aggravate acne.

What's Ahead

Attacking acne at the source is one goal of present-day researchers. They are investigating the use of topical medications that will curb oil gland activity without affecting the sex organs or producing any systemic side effects.

Actually, only so-called free androgens can enter oil glands and cause problems, and only one to two percent of the circulating androgens belong to this group (wreaking havoc way out of proportion to their numbers). The rest are bound to a special liver-based protein called ABG (androgen-binding globulin), which renders them inactive and unavailable to skin and hair cells. (Once the free-wheeling androgens come into contact with the target cells, heredity determines whether their impact will be moderate, severe, or nonexistent.)

There are new experimental anti-androgen drugs that promise to step up the body's supply of androgen-scavenging ABGs, block the conversion of weak androgens to strong ones (testosterone to dihydrotestosterone), or curb androgen's effects on target cells.

Though these developments are still on the drawing board, some researchers predict a chemical breakthrough in acne treatment before the decade is over. Right now they are exploring the safety and practicability of these newest ideas.

Finding a Dermatologist

Whether your case is moderate or severe, nothing will determine how fast or completely your condition improves as much as a solid, trusting relationship with your doctor. Often this is the crucial "missing link" in many otherwise sensible treatments for acne.

Ideally your doctor should play the roles of advisor and confidant at the same time. He should educate you about the real causes of acne and dispel myths (if you haven't already read this book to the end), reassure you that your pimples are not the result of failing to wash often enough or indulging in the wrong foods or harboring negative thoughts or masturbating. The doctor should also carefully record your acne history, noting such details as how and when the acne began and the patterns it shows (for example, whether you experience flareups during certain times of the year or periods of stress), your routine living habits, and any medication you are taking. (For example, a woman with severe, stubborn acne could not be given oral antibiotics because she was already taking drugs containing sulfur for a digestive-tract ailment. The two medications are known to conflict; besides, a compound like tetracycline might have aggravated her intestinal problem. This was a very vital piece of information for her doctor to know. He then compensated by designing an especially aggressive combination of topical treatments to eliminate her acne.)

Your doctor should always be sensitive to your doubts and fears regarding the treatment and willing to explain just how his approach will work (preferably with clear written and oral instructions), how long it will take, and what you should expect.

What you are responsible for is conscientious cooperation and follow through: disclosing enough accurate details about yourself, observing instructions, and asking questions if directions are unclear. This can help your doctor cure your problem in the safest, most effective way possible.

A sixteen-year-old boy with severe cystic acne believes the patient is responsible for ninety-nine percent of the result. "One should be a reliable team player," he observes, "carry out instructions such as when to take an oral antibiotic, for example, so that it's not counteracted by what you eat. Make sure your doctor gives your medication enough chance to work," he adds, "and yet is flexible enough to switch regimens when you're not getting the best results. Above all, be sure he spends enough time with you."

"I found some doctors too pampering and soft-pedaling," another patient complains. "They didn't seem to take my situation seriously enough. I was even treated right through my makeup. No one bothered to take it off to see how I really looked." Other doctors never encouraged or praised her for her efforts: "No one seemed to take notice of my progress or to be sympathetic about my little nagging anxieties. It was the doctor who finally stripped away all my layers of coverup, who was unblushingly direct about my condition and my treatment, that I ended up staying with until my acne was under control."

This patient's advice is to find a doctor who "sits down and talks to you about what your life is all about" before imposing any medication or course of action. "I once had very erratic, very disorganized eating and sleeping habits," she recalls. "The doctor who cleared my acne advised me to pace myself better all around and find more time for myself, so I could take proper care of my skin. This helped reduce daily stress and counter my negative self-image, both of which had been undermining my progress all along."

"I think your mind has to be an ally to your body for any treatment to work," another patient notes. "After my very first visit with the doctor who eventually cured me, my skin may still have looked the same, but I felt so confident and hopeful that I think half the battle was won right there and then. This doctor was compassionate, patient, and a good ear. He took the time to listen to my story and educate me about my treatment. I could just tell he knew what I had been going through. He seemed so interested, as if he were hearing all about acne for the very first time. His concern and encouragement made me believe in the therapy and trust his advice, and that helped guarantee the final result."

Sometimes, when an acne problem is especially severe and persistent, the family may be partly to blame. Parents, close relatives, and spouses can unwittingly sabotage efforts by being overly critical or impatient. Others can make comments that are grossly insensitive. Fathers call their sons "zit face" or ask them why they look so dirty and do not take better care of themselves. Unfortunately many people misguidedly hurt others with their comments and actually exacerbate the problem. When confronted with any serious or lingering case, an alert physician should ask searching questions about family attitudes.

The best doctor-patient relationship is direct, private, one to one. For example, an adolescent is not likely to cooperate with any dermatologist who says, "I'm going to tell your parents everything that goes on here at these sessions. They and I are going to participate in (or direct) your treatment." Of course, if a doctor works closely with his patients and earns their trust and respect, most of the time the family need not become involved at all. On the positive side, individual family members can be enlisted to offer encouragement and support.

Where and how should you conduct your search for a good dermatologist? A recommendation, particularly from a satisfied relative or friend who had a problem similar to yours and whose judgment you respect, is one place to start. A family doctor is another trustworthy source. If you do not have a personal physician and do not know anyone who has consulted a dermatologist, consult the department chairman at a local university or medical center or ask a county medical society or university hospital for a list of names. Do not hesitate to find out a doctor's credentials, whether he did his residency at a reputable medical center, and how many and what kinds of cases and procedures he handles every week.

A multivolume guide called *The Directory of Medical Specialists,* available in the reference rooms of most large public libraries, is another source of qualified practitioners in your area. Try to find a dermatologist affiliated with a medical school and/or well-established hospital. To have staff privileges, he is obliged to have satisfied some stringent requirements and to have attained a certain level of experience and expertise, and his hospital connection will ensure that you will be sent to a good medical facility should you require special care. Also, make sure your choice is board-certified, which means highly trained, with a passing grade in a competitive exam, and one who is a fellow of the American Society for Dermatologic Surgery.

Ask about fees at the outset; many doctors are willing to make adjustments for those whose needs outweigh their ability to pay or to refer you to less expensive but equally competent colleagues. Remember, high price is no guarantee of expert, personal care.

Once you have narrowed your choices, consult with several physicians before making a final decision. Make sure you receive satisfactory answers to the following questions. Is the doctor willing to talk about the possible side effects or drawbacks of your treatment? Can you call him or his office during out-of-hours emergencies? Will he tailor a regimen just for you or does he have one standard treatment for everyone? (Ideally a doctor should consider each patient a new, "original" case and regard himself as an investigator, ferreting out important clues and conducting a thorough search.) If possible question the doctor's patients. Does the doctor answer their questions adequately, encourage them to voice their fears or doubts? Does he notice and comment favorably when patients' condition improves, giving them the boost they need to continue? Do the patients know the names of the drugs they are taking and the lotions they are using, and how and when they should be used for best results?

Keep in mind that getting your acne cleared is a two-way proposition, as one patient notes. "Both sides, doctor and patient, have to contribute to the outcome by being open and cooperative."

Your Own Worse Enemy?

Sometimes, even after finding the best medical care, patients become their own worst enemy. As doctors can testify, a distorted self-image can pose a very real obstacle to people seeking treatment. Some people emphatically deny to themselves that a skin disorder exists at all, while others absurdly exaggerate their condition. In other cases, patients accurately size up their problem but have a curious stake in preserving the status quo.

In spite of their protests to the contrary, many people have something to gain by clinging to their acne. It gives them a perfect excuse for social failure or rejection, an acceptable reason for avoiding interaction with the opposite sex when that looms as an overwhelming test of their personal worth. Others feel their condition is a way of attracting attention, love, or sympathy, which they fear would be abruptly withdrawn if they were suddenly cured.

For this reason it is not uncommon for patients to be enthusiastic about their treatment and supremely cooperative with their doctor at the very beginning, then, unaccountably, stop taking medication or break appointments as soon as their condition shows signs of improvement. In other cases, patients become involved in an unhealthy hostile-dependent relationship with their physician. Outwardly they accept his treatment, but proceed to thwart it in subtle ways, accidentally "forgetting" to take their prescription drugs or deliberately misusing them.

Sometimes a patient's family feels (unconsciously) threatened by the prospect of a cure—perhaps they fear the patient will not need them as much once the disorder clears—so they undermine their loved one's efforts by chiding him for being overly serious or conscientious about the treatment or raising doubts about the doctor's approach.

Beware of these hidden enemies to your recovery, both in yourself and in others.

Acne Quiz

By answering the following questions you can help your doctor pinpoint the source of your acne and decide the best course of treatment.

1. Is your face dry, oily, or normal?

2. Is your hair dry, oily, or normal?

3. How often do you shampoo your hair?

4. Do you use anything on your hair for grooming?

5. How often do you wash your face daily? With what soap? Do you scrub or wash gently?

6. Do you use Noxzema, cold cream, suntan lotion, night cream, moisturizer, cleansing cream, makeup, baby oil, other creams? Do you use a water-base or oil-base makeup?

7. Do you use hand cream?

8. Do you sit with your hands on your face?

9. Do you wear a helmet, chin strap, backpack, shoulder pads? Do you weight-lift or put your hands on your face a lot?

10. Do you take any of the following medicines?

iron	INH
B$_6$ (pyridoxine)	Dilantin
B$_{12}$	phenobarbital
lithium	birth control pill
cortisone (prednisone, decadron, etc.)	

11. Have you given birth or stopped taking the birth control pill in the last year?

12. Does tension or stress, chocolate or any food, perspiration, sun exposure, lack of sleep, menstruation, or shaving worsen your acne?

13. Do you work in contact with grease (fast food, cars, machines, etc.)?

14. Are you exposed to any chemicals during your normal day?

15. Do you use cortisone creams on your face, hands, elsewhere?

16. What medicines have you taken for acne recently?
    antibiotics (by mouth, on skin)   zinc
    Retin-A (type)   drying lotions
    benzoyl peroxide lotion   special soaps
    liquid nitrogen, dry ice, ultraviolet light
    cortisone pills or injections
    hormones
    What has helped?

17. Do you plan to get pregnant soon?

18. Do you use an ultraviolet light or sunlamp at home?

19. Do you ski?

20. Do you pick or squeeze your bumps?

CHAPTER 6

HOW TO ERASE ACNE SCARRING

Until recently physicians hesitated to treat acne scarring until every last pimple had been cleared. No longer. Thanks to a number of new (or more refined) techniques, both problems can often be tackled at once before the disease has run its course. The immediate visual improvement results in a tremendous psychological lift. When people see themselves looking better, they are more apt to follow their treatment regimen with care.

Everyone has a unique combination of scars, and very often more than one approach is needed to achieve the smoothest possible look. The color and texture of your skin and the extent and location of your scars also help determine what methods your dermatologist will choose. Consider the following options.

Collagen
For soft, craterlike pits and depressed linear scars, collagen implants derived from cow skin are the newest solution. Collagen, a form of protein, is a natural component of skin, bone, tendon, and other building block tissues that hold the body together. Commercially known as Zyderm, this highly purified bovine product has been recently approved by the Food and Drug Administration for use by highly trained dermatologists and plastic surgeons. Laced

with an anesthetic, it is injected with a fine-gauge needle into depressed skin tissue to elevate the area, smooth out the scar or defect, and replace the missing soft tissue. Unlike silicone, collagen eventually becomes a natural, living part of your body, complete with nourishing blood vessels and indistinguishable from the rest of your skin.

Since some of this soft white gel is actually absorbed into the body, your doctor will have to compensate for this by injecting enough to raise the scar above the level of the surrounding skin. When swelling and (possibly) slight bruising subside in six to twenty-four hours (sometimes longer), he can then decide how much more will be necessary for a uniform look. Generally only two to six treatments, on an outpatient basis, are required to achieve maximum correction.

Before treating you with Zyderm, your physician should perform a preliminary patch test to make sure you have no preexisting allergy to either the bovine material or to the anesthetic, xylocaine. (A small amount is injected into the inner forearm, followed by a thirty-day waiting period.) If dermabrasion is also being considered, collagen should be implanted either three months before or three months after dermabrasion for best results. You are not a candidate for collagen implants if you are pregnant or suffer from any active skin inflammations or autoimmune disorders, such as rheumatoid arthritis, ulcerative colitis, myasthenia gravis, or any other mixed connective tissue diseases. People who have been treated with silicone are now also considered candidates for collagen therapy.

Steer clear of direct sunlight for at least several months after collagen treatment. This is recommended as a precaution, since physicians do not know whether ultraviolet radiation will affect the chemical structure or texture of the implant or impair the outcome in any way.

After nearly six years of thorough testing by selected dermatologists and plastic surgeons, Zyderm has recently obtained Food and Drug Administration approval for more widespread use. Of the nearly twenty thousand people treated so far, over eighty percent have reported highly favorable results, and intermittent swelling for about two months was the only serious complication reported. The scars that respond best to Zyderm are soft and pliable; hard or very recent scars or those with very distinct margins, such as some pockmarks or deep "ice pick" holes, are difficult to correct with this technique. (See Chapter 8 for more information on collagen.)

Note: Only physicians with advanced training in soft tissue contouring or skin anatomy should administer the Zyderm implant. Make sure your doctor has these credentials.

Punch Grafts and Excisions

Scars with distinct margins are better served by punch graft replacements. The defect is removed with a small, light cookie cutter type of instrument and replaced with a tiny, smooth circle of skin taken from behind the ear. The plug fits right into the place of the newly excised scar, thus raising the skin level. For best cosmetic results, a doctor might smooth out the edges of the freshly fitted skin with electrodesiccation (very mild, short bursts of electric current applied with a needle). This relatively simple procedure can be performed with the patient under local anesthesia in an upright position.

Sometimes a depressed scar can be improved by simple punch elevation. The plug containing the scar is raised by the same instrument to a level flush with the surrounding skin. Both excision and elevation can be performed in a well-equipped doctor's office.

A few isolated but sizable, sharp, well-defined scars may be treated with individual excisions. First a large, deep crater is cut out, then the skin is stitched back together, leaving a smaller, less visible defect in its wake. The resulting mark can be almost undetectable if the original scar lies in a wrinkle or fold of skin. Remember, if a scar is not sharply outlined, it may respond well to collagen.

Cryosurgery
This is another approach to shallow or raised scars, involving the use of liquid nitrogen or another freezing agent to peel away selected areas of the face. By unblocking the follicles or glands affected by acne, this sprayed-on "controlled frostbite" treats active acne at the same time as it evens out pigmentation and helps camouflage scarring, rounding off the edges of shallow depressions and lightening the flat, discolored patches of burned-out lesions.

Dermabrasion
This in-office procedure consists of sanding down the outer skin; it is the treatment of choice when scars are widespread. Dermabrasion may take from twenty minutes to an hour or longer, depending on the skill of the operator and the area to be treated. The doctor administers a local anesthetic such as xylocaine, preceded by a mild sedative if you are overly tense. Next the face is numbed with a special freezing agent, which turns the surface rigid and hard, ready for sculpting. Then a high-speed mechanical abrader, fitted with a stainless steel wire brush or diamond-surfaced wheel, is applied to the entire face from hairline to jaw, or occasionally just to dime-sized areas. (The wire brush generally gives superior results.) Superficial layers of skin are removed and with them the shallowest remains of acne. The procedure can be repeated several times to improve more deeply pitted sections.

If scars are also treated with punch grafts, collagen, or silicone, a dermatologist may have to perform a full-face dermabrasion only once or twice. A second dermabrasion may be done from six to twelve weeks after the first, but it is better to wait six to twelve months to see how much the natural healing process will reduce remaining scars. Dermatologists try to avoid spot dermabrasions, because the treated skin may grow back noticeably lighter or darker than its surroundings, posing a real cosmetic problem.

Dermabraded skin remains raw and reddened for awhile,

looking sunburned for at least several weeks. Normally a protective, though none too attractive crust forms over the moist, oozing skin (like the scab of a scraped knee), which usually falls away within seven to ten days. However, splashing with tepid water frequently throughout the day will help prevent or minimize the crusting effect. Wash your hands or put on latex gloves before dousing your face. Some physicians provide a sterile saline solution to use in place of tap water for the first few days. If the splashing method is repeated diligently over three to four days, it will stop blood serum from draining and will dry out the skin, making it far less likely that thick crusts will form. Protective ointments can be then applied to smooth and soften the skin and curb excessive dryness.

Expect some slight throbbing and swelling, too, especially if skin has been planed around the eyes and neck. To minimize fluid buildup, sit or walk about as much as possible and sleep with several pillows for the first few nights or upright in a comfortable chair. You will probably feel better on the day of the operation than on the following few days, so if you have traveled from a distance, return home immediately or remain in the doctor's vicinity for at least four or five days. If you have the least touch of vanity, you will probably choose to stay out of the limelight for about ten days. Women can wear prescribed makeups and men may shave by the sixth to eighth day. Perhaps the most important postoperative advice is avoid the sun completely or use a total sunblock cream for at least six months, because the pigment cells of the face are temporarily altered by this process and the planed skin can be penetrated more readily by ultraviolet rays.

No elaborate preparations are required for a dermabrasion. Simply get a good night's sleep, the amount you require to feel well relaxed and refreshed. Avoid drinking much alcohol or any other stimulating beverage the night before. Eat a normal, leisurely breakfast. Arrive at the doctor's office with freshly washed hair and face (free of makeup or closely shaven) or other area to be treated. If possible, bring someone with you.

Sharp-edged acne scars that cast shadows and give the skin a moonscape look can be blunted with this technique. Raised scars are sanded down while indented ones blend in better with surrounding skin. In general, those scars that look better after the skin is manually stretched will improve dramatically after a single dermabrasion. If done properly, dermabrasion can even be adjunct therapy for active acne. While it is rarely used as a primary treatment today, it removes cysts, drains infected lesions, and alters the openings of sebaceous glands.

In any case, the procedure requires deft, experienced hands and good postoperative care. If skin is abraded too superficially, improvement may be minimal; if too many layers are removed, mottling or bleaching and scarring may result. If collagen and dermabrasion treatment are both considered necessary, these two procedures should be spaced at least three months apart.

The darker your skin, the greater your chances of discoloration and splotchiness. Blacks and Asians should be especially wary. The former run the risk of keloids (thick raised scars) and the latter of erratic and very persistent pigment problems. Bleaching creams or peeling preparations and even skin grafts can help restore color if it does not return on its own.

Some people react to dermabrasion with temporary outbreaks of milia (small white raised bumps) as the skin gradually heals. Do not pick at these or you will induce permanent scarring. They can be removed easily and painlessly with an electrical or surgical needle. To reduce ordinary soreness, dryness, or itching after bandages are removed, dab the skin with cotton soaked in equal parts of milk and ice water or apply a hydrocortisone lotion recommended by your dermatologist or pharmacist.

Because of the possible complications, your dermatologist may recommend abrading a nickel-sized test area of skin beforehand to see how you react.

Chemical Peeling

This technique involves brushing the entire face or selected parts of it with chemicals of varying strengths (typically, trichloracetic acid or buffered phenol) to slough away outer layers of skin and eliminate shallow scars. The chemical solution is spread with a cotton-tipped applicator or soft brush and left on for about a minute, then taped. Chemical peeling does not penetrate as deeply as dermabrasion, and the outcome is not as easy to predict and control. Uneven pigmentation is more likely to result from chemabrasion than from dermabrasion.

Fair skin responds best to both dermabrasion and chemical peeling, whereas olive, black, and oriental complexions may become severely discolored (possibly a permanent condition).

You will probably want to avoid appearing in public for a week to ten days after treatment. For the first day or two your face will be bandaged with tape; the skin remains dark pink for several days after its removal. Throbbing and swelling will cause some discomfort but can be reduced by your sitting up or walking about as much as possible.

Crusts may develop but can be prevented or minimized by your frequently splashing your face with tepid water throughout a four- to five-day period. If crusts do form, your physician will give you special instructions on how to wash them off at some time after the third day. A faint pink glow will linger for one to six weeks, the degree depending on your complexion and skin tone. Men and women may wear a prescribed cosmetic makeup while the skin is healing, and men may shave on the fifth or sixth day.

Operations on small sites on the face, eyelids, or mouth may not require more than one or two days' absence from work or social activities.

In all cases, however, avoid both direct and reflected sunlight for at least several weeks after the bandages are removed. Even a few seconds of exposure may alter pigmentation and mar the results. Protective sunblocks and screens recommended by your physician should be lavishly applied when you return to a normal schedule.

Final results are best judged after at least six months, when all swelling has subsided and the skin surface is fully exposed. (A puffed-up face often looks smoother than it actually is.)

Silicone

Minute amounts of purified silicone, an inert liquid, can be injected into shallow scars. The silicone creates activity within cells which causes the production of a natural collagen over a period of one to three months. The number of injections required to correct an individual scar depends on how much collagen is produced by the process. This is generally a safe procedure, since fibrous material forms around the silicone droplet, preventing it from breaking loose.

There is an optimal way of correcting or camouflaging every kind of scar. Dermabrasions are often done in combination with chemical peels, collagen or silicone injections, and punch grafts. Raised scars can be repeatedly frozen; excess tissue can be electrically singed away; they can be shaved off at skin level with a razor-like blade or cut out, the remaining skin being sutured or left to heal under bandages. Another possibility is to inject them with minute amounts of corticosteroids, which reduces collagen formation and flattens them out (producing the opposite effect from injections of silicone or collagen). Keloids are treated by injections of corticosteroids, cryosurgery, or a combination of both. They can also be excised at the base and injected at three- to four-week intervals. The corticosteroids are given in a more concentrated dose than those used to treat inflammatory acne.

Regardless of how scars are erased, follow-up care will hasten healing and keep discomfort to a minimum. All freshly treated skin is sensitive and easily irritated, so a good rule of thumb is to observe the guidelines for dry (fair) and sensitive skin offered in Chapter 2. Sunscreens under makeup are indispensable, especially for dermabraded and chemically peeled skin. The alternative is to have a very competent pharmacist or chemist add a sunscreen to the makeup.

Even after scars have been leveled and acne cleared, do not assume you can wear oil-based makeups and moisturizers with impunity. Since acne is never cured, only controlled, the conditions that allowed it to flourish in the first place can set the stage for trouble again.

As with any cosmetic procedure, expect to see only relative improvement. Silken-smooth perfection can never be guaranteed, nor is it necessary in this age of sophisticated coverups. Remember, too, that some scarring will fade automatically over the years. Your dermatologist may be able to predict which will disappear without outside help.

CHAPTER 7

SUN: YOUR SKIN'S WORST ENEMY

If skin care had to be summed up in just five words, almost every dermatologist would advise: "Stay out of the sun"—a message most of us conveniently ignore. After all, a well-bronzed body is fashionable, healthy-looking, undeniably sexy. And an off-season tan is still a mark of affluence. At once a natural tranquilizer and gentle stimulant, the sun relaxes muscles, improves circulation, and restores flagging spirits. It can serve as an antidote for mild acne, asthma, and aching joints, help clear up psoriasis, and enliven a lackluster complexion.

But nothing accelerates aging more dramatically than exposure to ultraviolet radiation. Sun-dried skin is quick to develop fine lines and wrinkles. Worse, the sun inflicts deep tissue damage, causing collagen fibers in the skin to break down and lose their elasticity. Your skin cells record every single photon* they are exposed to from birth. Over the years the photons mount up, as if on a charge account. Eventually you have to pay a steep price in the form of coarse, leathery skin, weakened blood vessels, loss of tone and resilience, and greater susceptibility to skin cancer. Sunlight is also believed to trigger changes in white blood cells that may impair the function of the immune system, the body's natural defense against disease.

*unit of ultraviolet radiation

If you are still not convinced about the impact of sun, compare the well-covered parts of your body, such as the abdomen or undersides of your arms, with exposed areas—face, neck, back of hands. Or to get some idea of how sun, wind, and elements can weather skin, throw a colored fabric out on the lawn. Within weeks the dyes will fade, the texture will turn rough and scratchy, and the weave will stretch out of shape.

A tan is the body's built-in—though only partial—shield against sunlight. To protect itself, exposed skin prompts special pigment-producing cells called melanocytes to turn out more granules of melanin (brown/black pigment), which work their way from the lower layers of the epidermis to the surface. The melanin granules collectively filter out a good portion of ultraviolet light, but damaging rays still invade the living portion of the skin. All people, regardless of skin type, have the same number of melanocytes, but those with deeper-toned skin produce more and larger melanin granules, which remain separate and intact when they migrate up ward instead of clumping together and disintegrating as they do in fairer skin. Besides tanning, the body also defends itself against the sun by thickening the skin's protective outer layer or stratum corneum, which gives chronically sun-exposed skin its leathery toughness.

Ultraviolet radiation comes in two varieties: short, intense burning rays called UVBs and slightly longer, milder, yet more deeply penetrating tanning rays called UVAs. The former prevail between the hours of 10 A.M. and 2 P.M., when the sun's power is at its peak. Besides painful burns, UVBs are responsible for pre-malignant growths, such as actinic keratoses, basal and squamous cell cancers, and the more severe malignant melanoma, all of which make their first appearance in the upper and middle layers of the epidermis. UVB damage to the cell-producing part of the epidermis and nearby pigment cells results in blotchy, uneven color—mottled, freckled, mole-marked skin.

A substantial portion of the UVBs reach into the dermis, or deeper layers of skin, too, where they undermine its supporting collagen fibers (which gradually lose their natural body and flexibility). Furthermore, UVBs damage blood vessel walls, impairing circulation. The diminished blood supply starves the collagen of vital nourishment and eventually makes skin more susceptible to extremes of heat and cold. UVBs also cause an important skin protein called elastin to form in an abnormal way. Excessive amounts of this raw material are produced but the quality is poor; it is flaccid, flabby, shapeless, and without its natural "spring." The visible results are loose, sagging folds and nubby, yellowish patches on the surface of the skin.

While less concentrated, the UVAs (once thought to be harmless) are actually more insidious, since they bombard us morning, midday, and late afternoon all the year round. Their presence intensifies the harmful effects of UVBs. They are also directly responsible for phototoxic reactions— the increased susceptibility to sunburn that accompanies the intake of certain drugs or medications, such as antibiotics, diuretics (water pills), antihistamines, tranquilizers, and oral contraceptives. The more deeply probing UVAs are about ten times more prevalent than UVBs during intense daylight hours. Their destruction is continual, subtle, and stealthy, and accomplished without a single trace of redness.

Your skin's color and thickness help determine how susceptible you are to the ravages of sun. The more natural pigment and layers you have, the greater your protection, but no skin is sun-resistant. In fact, people with a black, brown, or olive complexion may be overconfident about their inborn tolerance and fail to take the right precautions. Remember, your face and body do not have to burn outright to suffer permanent damage. Contrary to myth, no tan is beneficial. Even lightly toasted skin has been bombarded by enough radiant energy (those inescapable UVAs) to help age it prematurely. Besides, there is a considerable delay between what happens to skin inside and what is visible on the surface. Put another way, sunbathing in youth is a time bomb that may not go off for decades.

Almost every line, fold, and furrow etched in an over-forty face can be traced to a normal, outdoor-loving childhood.

Sunlight is a major *preventable* cause of wrinkling, and the sooner you prevent it, the better. In fact, if you slathered your face and body carefully with a good sunscreen from the very first year of life and never overexposed yourself, you would probably look little different at middle age from the way you looked at twenty. Wiser than they knew, our great-grandmothers preserved their porcelain-smooth looks with wide-brimmed hats and parasols (and by taking the sun in small doses). Today, chemicals which block, absorb, or scatter rays can be highly effective ways of slowing down the clock. To work, however, such protection should be a daily, year-round concern; exposure does not begin and end at the beach. Count strolling and shopping along city streets, working in the garden, and relaxing in the park at lunchtime as sun-filled minutes and hours that will ultimately take their toll. Even time spent driving or sitting indoors near windows should be added, since UVA rays can penetrate ordinary window glass.

Most sunscreens are now rated numerically according to a special scale called the SPF (Sun Protection Factor). The numbers, generally ranging from 2 to 15, are printed on the label. They indicate how much time you can expose yourself before the very first blush of sun (or pale pink) appears. When referring to unprotected skin, scientists call this the minimal erythema dose or MED. Normally, fair, easily freckled skin without a sunscreen will take about fifteen minutes to turn a faint red, whereas olive skin may take thirty to forty minutes, and very black skin, up to two hours.

Think of the SPF on the sunscreen label as a simple multiplication table telling you how many times longer than your MED you can stay out before starting to burn. Say you have a medium tone skin, which makes your MED or minimum safety time about twenty-five minutes. If you use a product with an SPF of 6, you can bask in the sun up to 150 (6×25) minutes, or two and a half hours, provided you have followed instructions and reapplied after swimming and sweating. Then you will have to reapply the product to maintain your advantage. Consistent daily use of a good quality formula will result in a gradual buildup of sun-fighting ingredients in the topmost layers of skin, thus enhancing your protection.

Sunblocks or physical screening agents such as titanium dioxide and zinc oxide, opaque materials that block and scatter light, act as mechanical barriers to both UVB and UVA rays alike. Thick, paintlike, and visible, they are usually worn by lifeguards and other people who spend long hours in the sun. While not cosmetically elegant, they are practical and effective when appearance is not at a premium. Commercial preparations such as A-Fil and RV Paque ointment are given a flesh-colored tint for more aesthetic appeal.

Most sun protectives are light, transparent lotions or gels that act by absorbing rays chemically. The best ultraviolet absorbers are PABA (para-amino-benzoic acid) or its derivatives and a group of compounds called benzophenones. Since the first soak up UVBs and the second UVAs, only a product containing both offers complete protection. (Remember, the lips, nose, and skin around the eyes should all be given an extra coat.) Some of the latest formulas are partly water- and sweat-resistant, so they do not need to be reapplied as often. Many contain moisturizers to hydrate skin and protect against aging dryness. Acting on the new notion that screening should be a year-round concern, cosmetic companies are now developing mascaras, eye shadows, foundations, and face makeups with sun-filtering agents.

No sunscreen should ever give you a false sense of security. Even the most potent products still allow a significant amount of solar radiation to reach the skin. And they offer no defense against either the visible or the infrared (heat) portion of the daytime spectrum. No one has yet determined the latter's long-term effects, but we do know that excessive heat readily penetrates the skin, contributing to blood vessel damage, changes in pigmentation, even heightened susceptibility to skin cancer. For example, skin cancers and dry skin problems proliferated in Europe during decades when central heating was virtually nonexistent and people often warmed themselves by sitting next to small coal fires. This suggests that radiation in the form of light is not the only hazard. Some scientists predict that future products will be developed not only to block untraviolet rays but also to absorb some of their heat.

Keep in mind that sunscreens work well in research laboratories because they are tested under controlled, ideal conditions. A more severe test is made when users are swimming energetically or playing aggressive tennis in a hot, humid environment. So it is always better to apply a product more lavishly and frequently than the instructions call for. (One thick coat of an oil-based lotion is roughly equivalent to two of a quick-drying gel.) Always apply the sunscreen evenly over dry, clean skin. Smooth on with one-way strokes. Do not rub it into your skin; rubbing may make it peel off. If if does, wash with soap and water, dry the skin, and reapply evenly.

If your skin is especially dry or sensitive, look for products containing PABA and benzophenones but no alcohol. Regardless of your skin type, sunscreens should always be used over moisturizer and under makeup. When at the beach, apply extra amounts to parts of the body that are usually covered up. These are particularly delicate and prone to burning because they have not built up any melanin barrier. Since lips contain virtually no melanin, women who do not wear lipstick and men should use an ultraviolet-absorbing lip pomade. (The darker shades of lipstick are the best protection.)

Occasionally some people prove allergic to PABA, which is chemically related to benzocaine. To test your reaction, apply PABA to a small area of skin for a day or so. If it turns out to be irritating, Padimate O and salicylates are good substitutes.

Researchers at the University of Nebraska Medical Center are developing a sunscreen (consisting of two salves) that can be applied at bedtime. The salves react together with proteins in the outer layers of the skin to change the ultraviolet receptivity of the skin by morning. The result is a protective shield that cannot be washed away by soap and water (and which need be reapplied only once every three or four evenings. When perfected, the product, designed originally for people who are overly sensitive to the sun, may be this decade's ideal sunscreen, becoming a natural part of our nightly ritual, like brushing our teeth.

Skin Types and the Sun

Sensitivity to the sun is most pronounced in a condition called albinism, which results from inadequate melanin in the skin. Without such an inborn shield, albinos are especially prone to the ravages of skin cancer, burns, blotches, and premature aging.

The Cuna Indians, who live about seventy miles from the equator, have no appreciable pigment, either. By the tender age of six, most show signs of solar (actinic) keratoses, rough, scaly-red, precancerous growths. By the age of fifteen, the majority have full-blown skin cancer.

The Celtic types, whose families come from Ireland, Wales, Scotland, Australia, and England, are another highly sensitive group. Their bodies do not manufacture enough melanin to produce any sun-blocking tan. They also have thin skin, more transparent than usual, and a marked tendency to freckle.

Regardless of what skin type you are, always apply a maximum protection sunscreen (15) and avoid switching to lower-numbered formulas as (or if) your skin tone darkens. Since even the most potent screens still allow solar rays to penetrate, you will tan, but you will tan more slowly. A well-known dermatologist suggests thinking of these sun-fighting gels and lotions as forming a kind of window screen or grating on top of your skin. The lower the SPF rating, the larger the holes and the more radiation can penetrate; the higher the number, the smaller the holes. But the barrier is never solid; a significant amount of sunlight invariably gets through. Remember, tanning is the skin's rather feeble defense against ultraviolet damage—and a visible sign that damage has already taken place.

Identify your sun quota by referring to the general descriptions below. Most sunscreens should be reapplied after swimming or sweating.

1. Very fair, thin-skinned, with light eyes and hair. Generally of Celtic, Scandinavian, or German origin. Never tans, may freckle profusely, burns very readily. If you are this type, your body was never meant to spend any length of time soaking up sun. Doing so is like going against your genetic grain, and results are guaranteed to be disastrous. Your MED is about 10 minutes. This means that with an SPF 15 sunscreen, you can stay out a total of 2½ hours (10×15 or 150 minutes).

2. Fair skin, with light eyes, often dirty blond or auburn hair. Burns easily, is very slow to tan (if at all). Your MED is about 15 minutes. This means that with an SPF 15 sunscreen, you can stay out a total of 3¾ hours (15×15 or 225 minutes).

3. Medium-toned skin, with light-brown eyes and hair. Can tan fairly well if exposed gradually, but will burn severely if not carefully screened. Your MED is about 20 minutes. This means that with an SPF 15 sunscreen, you can stay out a total of 5 hours (15×20 or 300 minutes).

4. Olive or yellowish skin, with dark brown or black

hair and eyes. Tans more readily than burns. Your MED is about 30 minutes. This means that with an SPF 15 sunscreen, you can stay out a total of 7½ hours. (15 × 30 or 450 minutes).

5. Light brown skin. Your MED is about 45 minutes. This means that with an SPF 15 sunscreen, you can stay out a total of 11¼ hours (15 × 45 or 675 minutes).

6. Black skin. Your MED is about 2 hours. This means that with an SPF 15 sunscreen, one application daily is probably sufficient.

Keep in mind that the time limits above are for sunscreens worn under ideal conditions, not when you are perspiring profusely or strenuously active, and applied carefully and thoroughly, not in haste. Also, other key variables should be considered when deciding how often to reapply your sunscreen, including the following.

Proximity to the equator: The closer you are to the tropics, the more intense the radiation. If you are medium-skinned, your burning time of 30 minutes will probably be reduced to about 15 minutes under such a concentrated sun.

Time of day: The hours between 10 A.M. and 2 P.M. (11 A.M. and 3 P.M. daylight time), when the sun's rays strike the earth at the most direct angle, pose the greatest risk of burning.

Time of year: During summer the sun's rays are the most powerful and direct, bombarding us with the greatest energy. Scantier clothing and longer days obviously add up to more exposure. Maximum protection is especially crucial at the beginning of the season, before you have had time to acquire a gradual tan.

Heat and humidity: The sun inflicts more damage in the presence of heat, a catalyst for the chemical reaction between ultraviolet radiation and skin. Since water is transparent to sunlight (only foam and whitecaps are not), you can get burned even if you spend all your time swimming under the surface. Damp or sweat-soaked skin burns faster than usual by permitting more rays to penetrate the outer layers. Wet clothing has the same effect.

Wind: Moving air can also intensify the ultraviolet onslaught. In a recent university study, mice exposed to both solar radiation and wind showed more underlying skin damage than those subjected to sunlight alone.

Reflective surfaces: Surfaces such as sand, snow, and concrete call for added SPF coverage, since they refocus scattered rays back toward the body. Thus, the shade of even the amplest canopy or umbrella affords relatively little protection at a sandy beach. Opaque, sun-absorbing surfaces such as grass and dirt are obviously more desirable.
   Note: Beware of sun reflectors. These collect and concentrate UV rays to a dangerous extreme and can accelerate damage greatly. The beaches of Estoril, Portugal, are lined with people stretched out on foil contraptions that look like the broiler pans used to cook chickens—and the results are virtually the same.

Oils: All oils, including baby oil and coconut oil, have a natural "broiling" effect, and so step up the rate at which you burn. They make skin more translucent, allowing sunlight to pass through more easily. (Hold up a piece of paper to lamplight before and after applying oil, and note the difference.) None offer any protection against either tanning or burning.

Drugs and Chemicals: Ingredients in aftershave lotions, astringents, perfumes, and colognes and antibacterial agents in medicated soaps and creams can make the skin more susceptible to burning, as can barbiturates, water pills, sedatives, antihistamines, blood pressure reducers, and oral contraceptives. If you are taking any medication at all, check with your doctor before exposing yourself to the sun.

Clouds: Do not be lulled by hazy, overcast days or cool offshore breezes. About seventy to eighty percent of the sun's burning power can penetrate even the thickest clouds.

Height above sea level: The higher the altitude, the less atmospheric buffer between you and the sun. For every 1,000-foot rise in sea level, the dose of ultraviolet radiation increases by five percent. So if you are escaping to a mountain resort, you will need more protection than if you are spending your days in a valley.

Much of the radiant energy approaching the earth is deflected by the oxygen in the upper atmosphere which is converted to ozone. The latter forms a natural layer of protection for the earth. So there is reason to be concerned about the fluorocarbons in aerosol sprays and emissions from supersonic aircraft, both of which are believed to strip away this ozone shield. Theoretically any decrease in ozone will hasten the rate at which the skin ages and heighten the risk of skin cancer.

Sunless Tans

For those with especially fair or sensitive skin, it may be wisest to look well-toasted without spending much time in the sun. This you can do by cheating with a synthetic tanning formula. These typically contain a sugar called dihydroxyacetone (DHA), which combines with amino acids (building blocks of protein found in the upper layers of skin) to stain the surface brown temporarily.

Synthetic tans do not wash off; they just fade gradually as the outermost cells are shed and the skin renews itself. Thus, they need to be reapplied every few weeks or so— only a minor price to pay for something that can prevent you from getting badly burned. Of course, never use a synthetic bronzer in place of a sunscreen; it provides absolutely no protection from ultraviolet rays. Applying a foundation several shades darker than your skin will also give you an attractive "tan."

Yet another way to fool Mother Nature is via the instant indoor tan. After basking nude for ninety seconds in the unearthly glow of purple bulbs lining a cozy cubicle (about the size of a large telephone booth), you can emerge with a coppery, head-to-heel tan indistinguishable from the tropical kind.

Recently the Food and Drug Administration required tanning salons to adopt stricter safety controls, such as better (automatic) timing devices, clear, well-placed instructions and warning signs on the dangers of overexposure, more careful screening and monitoring of customers, lamp shields to prevent injury, and obligatory use of protective goggles. But even with all these safeguards, a single dose provides four to five times the sunburning radiation of a noontime summer sun.

The store-bought approach is a still-booming phenomenon, perpetuating the myth that tanned skin is healthy and ultraviolet radiation another indulgence you can't do without. We strongly suggest you stay away.

Another sun-free tanner does not have to touch your skin at all. The Laboratoire Bioclinique of Montreal promises you a St. Tropez bronze after taking two to four capsules a day for at least two weeks. The active ingredients, canthaxanthin and beta-carotene, are already approved for use in the United States in limited amounts as red and yellow food dyes (found in butter, cheese, carrots, and sweet potatoes).

How does the product—known as Orobronze—work? Both compounds are absorbed by the intestines and deposited in the fatty tissues just beneath the skin, staining it a convincing coppery brown. After the initial build-up period, a half-dose taken every day should be enough to preserve the "tan."

The dyes have not yet been approved by the Food and Drug Administration for this purpose. At present Orobronze can be purchased only in Canada and Europe. While the capsules have been declared safe and effective abroad and can be bought over the counter, no one knows for sure whether systemic, continuing doses of these chemicals may do any long-term mischief. (The only side effect known to date is that the user's stools are red.) The real hazard, however, as with the liquid bronzers, is that the capsules may lull people into thinking they are shielded from ultraviolet rays. But Orobronze does not provide an adequate protective screen. Remember this limitation well. Since Canadian sales reportedly are booming, some observers predict that the "edible tan" may be on American drugstore shelves before long.

Sunburn

When skin is unprotected, ultraviolet burning rays can readily penetrate, tearing their way into living cells. The impact spurs an electrochemical change by splitting off parts of cells called free radicals. As their name suggests, these are highly volatile, indiscriminately destructive bits of matter that are released by the breakdown of fats (lipids) in the body and that can damage surrounding tissues.

When the process occurs in the skin, the result is a swelling and leakage of blood from tiny vessels in the skin—a process we call sunburn. Unprotected skin can burn within a matter of minutes, and even the most potent sunscreens are not reliable indefinitely.

A burn will peak within six to sixteen hours, so heed the following rule: Pink on the beach, scorched and suffering by late evening. If you begin to show pink, get out of the sun and take a cool bath quickly.

Suppose you miscalculate or fail to cover up? What can you do for relief?

For first degree sunburn—redness, pain, and swelling—use an over-the-counter hydrocortisone cream along with compresses made with either moist cornstarch or with a commercial oatmeal extract called Aveeno Powder (available in drug stores). Sprinkle it generously through a flour sifter into your bathtub as it fills with cool running water before you bathe. Or wrap ordinary dry oatmeal in cheesecloth or gauze, run cool water through it, discard the oatmeal, and apply the moist compress. Apply to sunburned skin every two to four hours. Ice, ice water, milk, and witch hazel also offer temporary relief, and some patients swear by the juice of a cucumber, slices of apple, or raw potato. Sleep on a water bed or air mattress or sprinkle talcum powder on your sheets thickly to minimize chafing and friction.

If you have a second degree burn, which causes the skin to turn a painful lobster-red and break out in blisters (involving a greater risk of infection), see your doctor. He may prescribe medications containing corticosteroids, indomethacin, or phenylbutazone. Whether your case is mild or severe, aspirin can reduce both the pain and inflammation. (Aspirin substitutes such as Tylenol offer no defense against swelling and redness.)

Skin Cancer

The same "free radical" damage triggered by ultraviolet rays also impairs cells' genetic blueprint, the crucial set of instructions the cells need to reproduce themselves exactly. This interference with cell formation and renewal can hasten aging; it also allows irreparably damaged cells to multiply, a condition that could lead to cancer.

Nearly all the 300,000 cases of skin cancer developed by Americans every year are believed to be sun-related. Not surprisingly, the disease, which takes a variety of forms, is most prevalent in the South and Southwest. But throughout the United States the number of skin malignancies has more than doubled within the last twenty-five years, presumably as basking on beaches and engaging in outdoor sports have become increasingly popular.

Some people are predestined to be vulnerable, particularly those who burn and freckle readily and who have blue or green eyes and fair skin and hair—notably Irish and other Celtic types. In fact, only South Africa and Australia have higher death rates for skin cancer than Ireland, even though it is located in a northern latitude and receives less than half the burning ultraviolet rays received by the other two countries.

The two most common and readily treatable cancers are the slow-growing basal and squamous cell varieties. As its name suggests, the former originates from the lowest part of the epidermis. Trouble starts when the basal cells, which ordinarily generate new tissue for the outer epidermis, start duplicating themselves erratically. This type of cancer rarely invades internal organs, although it will continue to grow relentlessly if left untreated. The second kind is slightly riskier, since it may travel (metastasize) to distant organs if neglected (though the chances are quite slim). With both kinds, chronically sun-exposed areas are frequent targets—face (including lower lip, eyelids, and ears), neck, forearms, and back of hands—though both cancers can arise elsewhere as well.

Basal cell cancers tend to have a shiny, translucent surface that feels smooth and waxy. They are usually flesh-colored to brown pearly papules, of almost any shape and size, raised along the edges and flattened or depressed in the center. Others have an orange-colored, gelatin-like appearance and are sometimes overlaid with a crust. Deceptively, basal cell cancers often flatten out and appear to heal without therapy, only to erupt again later on. Sometimes they bleed slightly, sometimes not at all, but because they disappear and are painless, patients often put off seeing a doctor. Unfortunately, recurring basal cell cancers are much harder to eliminate.

A squamous cell growth is typically a flesh-colored or reddish-brown nodule or wart, sometimes with scaling and ulceration. Like all tumors, these cancers are best treated early, when they are still small and confined, allowing for easier removal and superior cosmetic results.

A change in the size or color of a mole or sore is a signal that should send you to your doctor. Among the early warnings are raised, waxlike, pearly nodules and red, scaly patches with a sandy or grainy texture, a well-defined border, and possibly irregular shape. They do not blend in well with surrounding skin and may vary in size from one to four millimeters, though sometimes they are larger. Called solar or actinic keratoses or sun spots, these are a precancerous condition; if they are left untreated, there is a definite possibility that they may become malignant. Most common in pale-skinned, light-eyed people with a marked tendency to freckle, sun spots can be routed by topical chemicals such as 5-fluorouracil, which selectively colors the precancerous cells and causes the sun-ravaged skin to become raw and irritated. The abnormal tissue is permanently destroyed in the process while normal tissue remains intact.

Aside from chemical treatments, both tumors and premalignant growths can be frozen and peeled away by cryosurgery (in which liquid nitrogen is used to achieve a local frostbite and kill surface cells), blitzed with electric needles, or removed by curettage (scraping) or minor surgery. Sometimes a combination of methods is used.

The rarest, most serious (even potentially fatal) skin cancer, malignant melanoma, is not so directly sunlight-related, since it occurs as often on unexposed as on exposed areas of the body. (This suggests that certain genetic traits or environmental influences such as chemicals may be involved, possibly sometimes in combination with ultraviolet radiation. But melanoma does have a higher incidence in the South.)

One current theory suggests that melanoma strikes those who, normally confined indoors by their job, become overzealous in pursuit of the sun during vacations or weekend jaunts in the blazing Caribbean. Thus at highest risk are those who receive short-lived but intense exposure with little or no seasoning beforehand.

Malignant melanoma is so named because it originates in the pigment-forming cells of the epidermis. According to recent studies at the National Cancer Institute, people with a history of abnormal moles (a condition technically known as dysplastic nevus syndrome, or DNS) are particularly susceptible. In DNS, black or red-colored moles are larger, more numerous, and less regularly shaped than the normal kind. Scaling, flakiness, itching, and oozing are often present and breakouts occur all over, even on the scalp, where such growths normally do not take root. To diagnose the disorder before it leads to malignancy, people with numerous, unusually large, or oddly shaped moles are advised to examine themselves once a month for changes, have twice-yearly physical checkups, and keep sun exposure to a minimum.

Melanoma may appear as a flat, irregularly bordered, smooth-surfaced mole or stain, often red, brown, or black. Frequently larger than average and scaly or itchy, it may contain a notch and its color may change, subtly and slowly, turning bluish. Or it might be a mixture of colors, tan, brown, black, and reddish-pink. Of all the cancers, melanoma has the greatest tendency to spread to other parts of the body. Seventy percent of melanomas are called the superficial spreading type, which is most often found on the upper back of both sexes and on the lower legs of women. (For some reason, melanoma between the knee and ankle is nine times more common among women than men.) The disease has been on the increase steadily, even in northern climates, with the number of cases doubling every ten years since 1935.

Why do skin cancers of all kinds pose the greatest threat to the fair-haired and delicate-skinned? Here is a recent theory. A type of pigment called phaeomelanin has been found to be highly unstable in the presence of sunlight. When exposed to sunlight, this volatile substance readily bleaches and fragments; it undergoes chemical changes that may damage the reproductive ability of normal cells and so possibly pave the way for cancer. Since phaeomelanins are present in skin around the roots of fair hair and other parts of fair skin as well, they may help account for the higher incidence of skin tumors in light-skinned blonds and redheads.

A recent study at the University of California, Davis School of Medicine suggests that high levels of fat in the diet—particularly the polyunsaturated kind, found in vegetable oils—may promote certain forms of cancer by suppressing the body's immune response system. The growth of melanoma tumors was markedly accelerated in mice that were fed high polyunsaturated fat diets, the researchers found. Additional tests indicated that high levels of dietary fat in general, but especially the polyunsaturates, could inhibit the ability of certain cells in the animals' immune system, called lymphocytes, to kill injected cancer cells. Rather than promoting all types of cancer, the influence of dietary fat appears limited to tumors in certain tissues, such as the breast, colon, and skin.

Many health experts, concerned with reducing the risks of heart disease, have long advised Americans to lower their fat intake and substitute polyunsaturated vegetable oils for the more saturated fats in their diets. These latest findings, however, argue in favor of an overall decrease in fat in the American diet, ideally by at least twenty-five to forty percent.

Treatment

Most skin cancers can be treated right in the doctor's office. Curettage and electrodesiccation (blitzing with a fine-pointed electric needle) are probably the most common methods. These destroy little normal skin and are effective for small, primary tumors of the scalp, eyelids, lips, cheeks, ears, torso, and extremities. Other successful procedures are cryosurgery, radiation therapy, and surgical excision. All these give good cosmetic results and are relatively easy to perform.

Cryosurgery, or freezing with liquid nitrogen, is a quick, highly effective, painless, and inexpensive treatment for growths on the cheek, nose, lip, ear, trunk, arms, and legs. It is well suited for tumors with sharply defined outlines, especially those on the eyelid or nose, areas where other methods have specific drawbacks. For example, curettage and electrodesiccation are awkward to perform in such places, so cosmetic results may not be as satisfactory. Cryosurgery is also an ideal option for older patients who are taking anticoagulant (blood-thinning) drugs or who have to avoid surgery for other reasons. It is not the best choice, however, for tumors that lie on the tip of the nose or in the nasal creases. The nose may be noticeably notched or scarred after treatment, while cancers lying in the nasal folds are likely to recur if this method is used.

Cryosurgery can also cause a bleaching effect (hypopigmentation) on skin or erythema (swelling and redness) on certain sensitive parts of the face, especially near the eyes.

Surgical excision has the advantage of removing a specimen for closer inspection and is a one-step process. It does require anesthesia and carries a minimal risk of nerve or artery damage, as does any surgical procedure.

Radiation is often a less intimidating method psychologically and leaves tissue intact. However, it may accentuate scars and also cause temporary hair loss (alopecia areata). Normal surrounding tissue must be properly shielded to avoid unnecessary exposure. Also, radiation must be administered over several visits and is not always effective on tumors of the arms, legs, and upper body.

Right now scientists are working on the possibility of photo-radiation therapy. Ideally this would be a drug that is attracted only to malignant tissue, soaks up a wavelength of light that is not absorbed by normal skin, and has no systemic toxic effect.

One such agent under study today is called hematoporphyrin. Given intravenously, it seeks out and is retained only in cancerous tissue, is absorbed by a wavelength of light that does not affect normal tissue, and can treat a variety of tumors effectively. In one recent trial, thirty out of thirty-five patients with basal or squamous cell carcinoma were successfully treated by this method.

For secondary tumors (recurring growths), the best method is a technique called Moh's chemosurgery. This is a time-consuming procedure that removes the cancer layer by layer. It requires highly trained hands and is reportedly the treatment of choice not only for recurring tumors but also for those that have spread to bone tissue, some types of malignant melanoma, and large or deeply invasive growths with undefined borders.

Malignant melanoma responds well to surgery. A simple removal of tissue is all that is required for superficial tumors, while deeper growths call for wider excisions, along with skin grafts or cosmetic reconstruction to cover the resulting scar. When the lymph nodes are also affected (in more advanced stages of the disease), doctors often resort to chemotherapy, immunotherapy, or both. The BCG vaccine is one immune-boosting agent under current investigation. So far several promising studies have indicated that BCG may slow down the advance of the disease and increase the survival rate.

One variety of the disease, called lentigo malignant melanoma, which often occurs in older patients and those with chronically sun-damaged skin, can be snuffed out with cryosurgery. Radiation therapy is not considered beneficial for melanoma.

Some synthetic forms or analogues of vitamin A, called retinoids, have been shown to prevent or shrink certain cancers in animals. Now trials of both oral and topical compounds are under way. One is retinoic acid, the chemical that has worked such wonders for acne (see Chapter 5). Compounds in pill form, similar to those designed for psoriasis and severe acne, are reported to be of value against basal and squamous cell cancer.

Remember, skin cancer, even melanoma, offers one advantage not granted by other malignant growths in the body: visibility to the naked eye. Let the advantage be yours; stay alert to all the signals.

The following guidelines from the National Cancer Institute will help.

HOW TO PREVENT MALIGNANT MELANOMA

These guidelines are intended for those at high risk of melanoma either because they have had a melanoma in the past or because they have atypical moles on their skin.

1. Melanoma can be cured if found early. You must watch for changes in your skin and see your doctor promptly if you have any questions.

2. Get to know your skin. Spend some time looking at your skin, learn what it looks like, where birthmarks and moles are located and what they look like. Don't forget the hard-to-see areas, too, especially the back, the scalp, between the buttocks, and the genital area. You should examine your own skin at least once a month. Begin with your face and scalp, and step by step, look closely at head, neck, shoulders, back, chest, arms, legs, etc.

3. Find a good doctor for your skin care. This doctor should know the importance of your family background and be willing to remove any changing skin lesions early. Your skin should be checked by this doctor at least twice a year for the rest of your life. Sometimes, patients will go through a time during which their moles are changing quickly and many new ones are found. During such times of "increased mole activity," moles should be watched with special care and doctor visits should be increased to every three months. Be certain that the doctor examines your scalp, as well as the rest of your skin.

4. Melanoma danger signs
   • Change in size of a mole: A sudden increase in size is of special concern; slow change is much more common.
   • Change in color of a mole: Also of special concern is the mixing of shades of red, white, and blue, or a sudden darkening of brown or black shades.
   • Change in mole surface: Watch for scaliness, flaking, oozing, erosion (as when a scab comes off), ulceration, bleeding; appearance of a nodule or bulging, mushrooming mass.
   • Change in how a mole feels to the touch: Getting either hard or lumpy.
   • Change in shape or outline of a mole: Finding an irregular, notched border where it used to be regular and smooth; sudden elevation of a surface that used to be flat.
   • Change in skin around a mole: Spread of pigment

from the edge of the mole into skin that used to be normal-looking. Finding redness or swelling (inflammation); development of satellite pigmentation (that is, nodules of pigmentation next to, but not a direct part of, a mole).

• Onset of new feelings or symptoms in a mole: Feeling itchy, tender, or painful.

• Sudden appearance of a new pigmented lesion in an area of skin that used to be normal.

5. Spend as little time in the sun as you can. Ultraviolet (UV) radiation from the sun is the major known causative factor for melanoma of the skin. Time in the sun should be reduced as much as you can.

• Avoid getting sunburned and do not try to get a "good tan."

• During periods of work or play in the sun, avoid prolonged exposure between the hours of 10 A.M. and 3 P.M. from May 1st through October 31st, when the sun is strongest. If you live south of 35°N Latitude (that is, south of a line that runs roughly between Charlotte, North Carolina, and Los Angeles, California), sun bathing between 10 A.M. and 3 P.M. should be avoided year-round. Remember that a lot of UV radiation can pass through clouds or be reflected from snow or water. Thus, sunscreens may be needed even on a cloudy day or in the winter.

• If you must play or work in the sun, apply the highest SPF sunscreens and/or blocks to your skin.

• When you are out in the sun, wear your hair long (to protect the back of the neck), use a broad-brimmed hat, long-sleeved shirt or blouse, and long slacks. It is worth noting that UV radiation can go through a single layer of thin cotton (such as a T-shirt) and produce a burn or tan on the skin underneath. Thus, for prolonged sun exposure, a sunscreen is needed in addition to lightweight clothing.

• Don't forget that sun lamps used for indoor tanning are also a source of UV radiation and should not be used. Both ultraviolet and X-ray treatments for acne or other chronic skin conditions should be avoided. Although the effects are probably not very large, it is probably wise to avoid regular, prolonged exposure to bare fluorescent lights (as in an office or the kitchen). A glass or plastic cover over the fluorescent tube will block the small amount of UV they release. Also, it is probably wise to avoid photo-chemotherapy treatment ("PUVA") for other chronic skin conditions.

• Changes in hormone balance may cause moles to change. Extra careful doctor checkups are required during adolescence and pregnancy. The use of hormone drugs, such as oral contraceptives ("The Pill") or estrogens for treatment of menopausal symptoms should be avoided, if possible. Again, the evidence on which this last suggestion is based is not very strong, but there is enough concern to make caution worthwhile.

• Don't forget: Nearly 100 percent of strictly defined early stage melanomas can be cured, but advanced melanoma is a very serious, potentially lethal disease. Careful, regular self-examination, combined with frequent doctor visits, will detect mole changes early, and many changing moles will thus be removed before melanoma develops at all. Also, those few melanomas that do occur will almost always be found early in their course, at a time when they can be cured by surgery alone. Minimizing UV radiation exposure and unnecessary hormone use will also decrease the chance of getting a melanoma.

6. Don't hesitate to write to the following address if these guidelines are not clear or for help in locating a good doctor in your area:

Mark H. Greene, M.D., or Mary C. Fraser, R.N.
Environmental Epidemiology Branch
National Cancer Institute
Landow Building, Room 3C-07
Bethesda, Maryland 20205
(301) 496-4375 [Phone collect]

Commonly Asked Questions
How do unusual moles differ from ordinary moles?

	Ordinary	Dysplastic (unusual) moles
Color	Uniformly tan, brown one mole looks much like all others	Variable mixture of brown, black, red/pink within a single mole; moles may look very different from each other
Shape	Round; sharp, clear-cut border between mole and surrounding skin; may be flat or elevated (bump)	Irregular border; may have notches; may fade off into surrounding skin; always a flat portion level with the skin, often occurring at edge of mole
Size	Usually less than 5 millimeters in diameter	Usually more than 5 millimeters; may be more than 10 millimeters
Number	Typical adult has 10 to 40, scattered over body	Usually more than 100, although some patients may not have an increased number of moles
Location	Generally on sun-exposed surfaces, above waist; scalp, breasts, buttocks rarely involved	Back most common site; may occur below waist and on scalp, breast, buttocks

Are unusual (dysplastic) moles cancerous?

Strictly speaking, unusual moles are not cancerous and most will probably never be; however, they represent a susceptible phase that may progress to cancer. Unusual moles undergoing changes in size, color, surface, shape, or outline may be a warning of melanoma danger.

Reprinted by permission of The National Cancer Institute, Bethesda, Md.

CHAPTER 8

FORTY PLUS AND STILL BEAUTIFUL

The French have observed that a woman is not truly interesting until her fortieth year. While their wisdom in matters of beauty and elegance is rarely questioned, many women (and men) regard the prospect of an "interesting" face with more despair than jubilation.

No doubt some people seem graced with smooth, moist, clear-toned skin well into their forties and beyond. But if you just hopelessly envy their natural good looks, you have not got the message. Heredity may offer an advantage—the darker and thicker your skin, the less perceptibly you age—but other influences are even more important. Maintaining youthful skin calls for continual preventive care. That means keeping your insides healthy, since your complexion may mirror almost any malfunction in that magnificent machine, your body. That means eating, sleeping, and playing well, and avoiding the environmental elements that prematurely season skin. Fortunately, for those who have abused their skin, both restoring and sculpting a face well worn by time is now more possible than ever, thanks to advances in dermatology and the artful use of cosmetics.

In order to stave off the visible signs of aging, you should understand something about the subtle yet all too obvious process first.

How You Age

Until gerontologists discover the so-called supergene that will unlock the secrets of aging, growing older remains inevitable.

The body's cells are continually reproducing themselves. Nesting within each of them is their secret code, the complex, coiled strands of DNA and RNA that contain the exact blueprint for continual self-renewal. Over time this code begins to get scrambled or misinterpreted (just like a message that passes along a long line of people). Both internal and external forces contribute to the confusion, including ultraviolet radiation, environmental toxins, viruses, free radicals (destructive internal molecules), even the body's own heat. The repair mechanisms that normally correct such errors begin to break down, like all machines subjected to constant use.

How does this apply to skin? Skin cells normally regenerate themselves on a regular basis as outer layers slough off and newer ones form beneath. Young skin renews its surface every three to four weeks; but by the time you are in your thirties and forties, the process can take twice as long, and the under layers are not as perfectly formed as they used to be. With fresher-looking cells stalled below, the complexion takes on a sluggish look and loses much of its tone and vitality. A dull, flaky film builds up as dehydrated, flattened cells accumulate near the top.

The slowly shed layers also have time to absorb more melanin (pigment) than usual from surrounding tissues, which may give older skin its telltale mottled look. At the same time, both sweat and sebaceous glands become less active, diminishing in number and size. Normally their secretions help form a protective coat that seals in moisture and shields the outer layers from damage by pollution and wind. With less fluid and oil to plump up cells, skin is no longer as smooth and supple, and the surface is more likely to dry and crack.

Think of aging skin as a house; the foundation starts to wear away and the supporting beams are fewer and more brittle; the stage is set for a major collapse. Thus, as you grow older, your entire body mass starts to shrink. Less collagen is produced, fluids dry out, bones and muscles lose tissue. However, since the overlying skin remains the same in extent, the excess simply begins to sag and crease. The remaining collagen becomes increasingly knotted or cross-linked with tough, elastic fibers, making other areas of the skin stiffer and less pliable. As the skin gradually loses its capacity to spring back, temporary character lines become permanently imprinted on the face.

As if this were not enough, blood vessels begin to decline in number, slowing down circulation and heightening sensitivity to heat and cold. Also, fewer beneficial hormones are delivered to skin cells, leading to a loss of subcutaneous (underlying) fat. The result is a hollowed-out appearance: The bone structure beneath becomes more visible and the skin less firm, especially around the eyes and cheeks.

Unfortunately, you do not have to be old chronologically to show such external marks of age. The skin's chief opponent is not the calendar but rather chronic sun exposure. Whatever time would accomplish on its own, the sun dramatically intensifies and achieves much faster. In fact, there is little reason why your skin should not retain much of its original baby-smoothness thoughout life, as long as you are always well protected from the sun's devastating rays.

The effects of ultraviolet radiation are cumulative and insidious, since the visible signs—wrinkling, dryness, dis-

coloration, broken blood vessels, sagging, thinning skin—
generally do not appear until ten or even twenty years after
underlying damage has already begun. And there is no
such thing as a healthy tan. The radiation that results in a
bronzed complexion is more than enough to damage the
tissues that support and shape the skin.

But even if you have overdone the sun in your early
years, it is never too late to slow down the aging process,
and the effects may even be partly reversible. With an
effective sunscreen, used every day regardless of season,
your skin can start to heal itself and counteract degenera-
tive changes. To ensure this, apply a good product as
regularly as you would brush your teeth; make it an unfailing part of your morning ritual unless you are planning to
remain entirely indoors.

Some very good evidence links smoking with premature
wrinkles, especially near the upper eyes. Precisely how
smoke may ravage skin it not yet understood, but it is
believed to result in the formation of chemicals called
aldehydes in the body which are very potent "cross-linkers."
Smoke is also known to deplete vitamin C, one requirement for healthy collagen. By constricting blood vessels,
smoking can fade and yellow even rosy, translucent skin.
And puffing and squinting through rings of smoke probably hasten creases around mouth and eyes.

Too much alcohol dilates blood vessels, leading to un-
natural flushing, blotchiness, even rosacea. It also converts
to skin-damaging aldehydes in the liver, dehydrates tissues
and interferes with the metabolism of vitamins, robbing
the skin of essential nourishment.

Constant on again, off again dieting and poor eating
habits can repeatedly stretch and contract the skin, breaking down the supporting fibers. The same applies to extremes of heat and cold, along with facial exercises (these
do anything but rejuvenate the skin).

Excessive washing and scrubbing, particularly with harsh
soaps and hot water, and an overheated or cooled environment can strip away the skin's natural protective layers

and essential oils, accelerating the appearance of fine, dry surface lines.

Everyone reponds to tensions and emotional upsets in a physical way, with clenched jaw, pursed lips, or furrowed brow. Stress causes the nerves to activate various facial muscles. As a result of constantly tensing and contracting, however, muscles tend to enlarge, and overlying skin must stretch to accommodate them. If it does this repeatedly (and especially if the collagen has already been damaged by sun), it will eventually sag and lose its shape, like an overworked rubberband, and develop a line or wrinkle. After a while, these become permanent and will not disappear even when underlying muscles are relaxed. Thus, the grimace, frown, scowl, and squint all eventually contort the features to produce the familiar crow's feet, forehead grooves, curved lines between the mouth and nose, and creases radiating above and below the lip.

Controlling those expressions assumed out of mindless habit rather than genuine spontaneity can help prevent such lines from deepening. Since they can persist even while you sleep, the nightly use of Scotch tape on crease-prone areas such as the forehead can help keep the skin smooth and wrinkle-free. Correcting astigmatism, myopia, and other eye problems can curb squint and resulting crow's feet.

Learning to defuse tensions and distribute stresses through total body movement is another way to relax the muscles of the face. Vigorous activity also provides a tremendous boost to circulation, which of course does wonders for your complexion.

Chronic loss of sleep will eventually show itself in a drawn, hollow-eyed look. Fighting off fatigue requires considerable effort. To make the body stay awake against its will, circulation is diverted from facial tissues to major muscles and organs; this drains the face of color and highlights under-eye circles by contrast. And the continued flow of adrenaline contributes to overwrought nerves. (That's why we turn irritable if deprived of sleep too long.) The result is frowning, squinting, and other strained expressions, which eventually become permanent lines if the habit persists.

Contrary to myth, skin generally looks its best earliest in the morning, because natural body fluid levels shift toward the head while we sleep. This fills out hollows and makes lines appear a bit less conspicuous. Excess swelling beneath and above the eyes and facial stretching caused by any accumulated body fluids—both more noticeable in an aging face—can be prevented by sleeping with the head in an elevated position.

Food and Moisture:
Age Prevention

Your skin needs special pampering when you are dieting if you aim to look youthful as well as slim. As pounds disappear, fat cells shrink, and already sun-damaged or overstretched skin can easily lose tone and resilience. Strive for a patient, two-pounds-per-week weight loss and staunchly ignore so-called miraculous crash plans. Unbalanced eating can leave your body vulnerable to stretch marks and ravage the face. And, as most people have ruefully discovered, pounds often return with compound interest when you go off a "quick slim" diet.

The best eating plan for youthful skin contains a well-balanced mixture of wholesome food in all categories (see Chapter 11). Take a vitamin supplement with minerals and keep liquid intake high, unless your doctor suggests otherwise. Adequate fluid keeps the skin moisturized from the inside and helps avoid drying and flakiness.

Gradual dehydration is inevitable with advancing age and steps up rapidly in such atmospheric conditions as overdry interiors and parched, windy climates. To combat dryness, plain tap water is the best solution. The skin's outer layer consists of overlapping cells, which under a microscope resemble the shingles of a roof. These external cells are naturally dry, but can absorb and retain water. With enough moisture in the outer layer, your skin swells and fills out slightly, camouflaging wrinkles and looking smooth and flexible. Every drop of fluid lost means a coarser appearance and texture to skin. So if daily care includes locking in natural moisture, you are well ahead in the aging game.

Dryness prevention consists of two phases. Replenish the water lost by evaporation by drinking five to six glasses of water each day (straight from the tap or the low-sodium bottled variety). The second phase, to be done several times a day, is external watering of your face and body. Apply emollient lotions or creams after your shower or bath while your skin is still slightly damp. This seals the water droplets in place and prevents their escape. In between, soak skin with cold compresses for a few minutes, then reapply moisturizer.

Trapping the moisture left on the skin with a thin layer of grease will allow each flattened outer cell to plump up attractively and protect your complexion against dry surface wrinkles. Look for products with such ingredients as urea, mineral oil, stearic or lactic acid, and lanolin. (See Chapter 2 for more on moisturizers.)

Treatments for Aging Skin: From Conservative to Radical

To revitalize skin and even reverse the effects of aging, dermatologists, plastic surgeons, and cosmetic chemists are continually refining and pooling their collective skills. Included in the present-day offensive against those dreaded wrinkles are chemical, mechanical, topical, and surgical solutions, used alone or in combination, depending on your skin type and age-related defects, among other variables.

A face severely damaged by sunlight or scarring may require a major mechanical overhaul, which is known as **dermabrasion**. The technique has been practiced for years, but a well-known colleague recently remarked that comparing today's methods with those of even a decade ago is like pitting the Concorde against the first airplane. Dramatic improvements in anesthesia and apparatus enable physicians to resurface the skin and remove fine wrinkles with greater precision than ever before.

After treatment, the newly planed skin, covered by medicated gauze or antibiotic ointments, swells and forms crusty scabs within one or two days; when these are shed, about ten to fourteen days later, the surface is pinker, fresher, thinner, and biologically younger. Even ten years later the skin will still look more youthful than it did before the procedure.

Dermabrasion can remove precancerous skin and eliminate the birthmarks that will not come out with bleaching creams or other methods. Deep scratches and upper-lip wrinkles also respond well to it. Results vary according to the depth of the lines or blemishes, the number of skin layers stripped away, and the number of times the procedure is repeated.

After dermabrasion, avoid excessive heat, cold, wind, and sunlight for at least several months, and always apply a maximum strength sunblock before venturing outdoors. The raw, reborn skin is highly sensitive to rough handling by the elements, and delicate surface capillaries may burst. Be prepared for some initially inflated results. Remaining lines and wrinkles, temporarily camouflaged by facial swelling, will reappear once the puffiness recedes—within about six months. (For more details on dermabrasion, see Chapter 6.)

Chemical peeling, or **chemabrasion**, accomplishes topically what dermabrasion does mechanically—peeling away the upper layers of skin. Mild swelling and redness follow for several weeks, after which the skin seems smoother and fuller, the lines less conspicuous, and freckles and age spots markedly lightened. You really cannot gauge final results for at least six months, since swelling obscures remaining lines and wrinkles.

Chemical peeling is probably most effective for the fine wrinkles radiating from the upper and lower lip. Results are lasting here, because the chemicals actually change the nature and texture of skin. When it regenerates after the superficial burn, the altered tissue is more wrinkle-resistant.

The major drawback is that it is hard to control and predict the effect of chemicals on skin; they cannot penetrate as deeply as dermabrasion, yet involve a greater risk of uneven pigmentation and possible scarring. Many physicians feel dermabrasion is safer, less painful, and gives a more cosmetically elegant result. (For more details on chemical peeling, see Chapter 6.)

Liquid injectable **silicone** acquired a deservedly bad reputation years ago because of its tendency to travel to other parts of the body. Now it is either encased in clear gel-like bags used to augment chins and breasts, or else injected in very small amounts to help replace tissue that has been lost because of age, disease, or trauma. A tiny droplet of silicone attracts fibroblasts that cluster around it while it actually builds new collagen cells. As a result, the silicone is bound and cannot escape. Some physicians have found it especially effective for filling out forehead furrows, vertical folds between the eyes, and the groove between lower eyelids and cheeks.

While silicone products and techniques have become ever more sophisticated, the newest breakthrough for wrinkles is **Zyderm**, a highly purified collagen protein taken from cow skin and processed into a form compatible with human tissue.

When it warms to body temperature, this injected bio-material is converted into a latticework of collagen fibers, much as individual threads combine to form a piece of cloth. The well-woven mesh becomes the base on which new tissue grows and multiplies. Cells and blood vessels move into the area, and it eventually takes on the qualities of normal connective tissue, with the texture and appearance of natural skin.

Like silicone, Zyderm is often used to fine tune the surfaces that cannot be directly helped by dermabrasion or cosmetic surgery. By raising the skin surface, collagen conceals a given line or wrinkle and also softens overlying skin. The best cosmetic results are achieved with the deep, curved folds between the nose and corners of the mouth, the horizontal grooves across the forehead, the vertical frown or scowl lines between the eyes (glabella), the hollows within the cheeks, and the folds that extend from mouth to chin—all hallmarks of aging that even a full face-lift cannot satisfactorily erase. (For more details on collagen, see Chapter 6.)

The area around the eyes is often the first to show signs of aging, because skin is thinnest there and thin skin wrinkles faster. Thin skin makes blood vessels more visible, so under-eye circles seem darker than surrounding skin. Fatigue accentuates the effect, because it drains the rest of the face of color.

A mild chemical peel, a prescription bleaching cream, or even cryosurgery can deal with excess pigment, while the groove between eyelid and cheek can sometimes be smoothed out with silicone or collagen.

In **cryosurgery**, the physician uses a probe containing liquid nitrogen or solid carbon dioxide (dry ice)—both exceedingly cold—to induce a local controlled frostbite that kills pigment cells on contact. Scabs form and are sloughed off within a week; the freshly healed skin generally grows back lighter. There is no need for an anesthetic because the freezing itself causes temporary numbness. No bandages are necessary, either, and you can walk out of the doctor's office just minutes after treatment. Some slight swelling and superficial peeling are usual aftereffects, and there might be some puffiness around the eyes.

Aside from being frozen, peeled, or bleached away, the individual specks and blotches, or age spots, that can mar an otherwise clear complexion can also be blitzed with a weak electric current through a needle (a simple technique called **electrodesiccation**). The swift jolt produces scaling and irritation, which will camouflage overpigmented or discolored areas. There is very little pain, but depending on the number of blemishes—and the squeamishness of the patient—the doctor may use a local anesthetic.

Despite their name, you do not necessarily have to be old to have age spots. These patches are flat, smooth in texture and brownish in color, and are usually found on the face, the "v" of the neck (upper chest), and hands. They are due to a high concentration of melanin and may be caused by overexposure to the sun. Unlike sun spots, however, they are completely harmless; there is no evidence that they are linked to cancer.

Store-bought bleaching creams containing hydroquinone, resorcinol, or salicylic acid can also lighten pigment after long, consistent use (sometimes months are required). Actually, such ointments work best on skin that has suffered pigment changes as a result of disease or injury; they are less effective when applied to normal healthy skin. Your dermatologist can provide a more potent, reliable, faster-acting preparation. Both prescription and over-the-counter products are believed to work by helping to suppress the skin's output of melanin and limit the number of pigment-producing cells. If you prefer to watch your spots fade away very slowly, be sure to buy a non prescription cream containing a sunscreen. If you go outdoors wearing a bleaching cream without a sun-protective agent, those age spots may actually get worse.

As for dilated ("broken") blood vessels, another sign of aging, electrodesiccation can blanch them instantly, eliminating the fine, spidery red lines around the nose, eyes, and cheeks, and even clusters of cherry-red papules called senile adenomas. The current coagulates the blood and breaks down vessel walls, which then disintegrate and disappear. Tiny scabs form, but these heal within a few days. Some barely perceptible scarring or small white spots may show up, and there is a small chance that the damaged capillaries will reappear. (Weakened blood vessels also respond very well to dermabrasion and chemical peel.)

Small skin tags or soft fibromas, tiny loose flaps of skin, may appear on the neck or armpit or around the eyes as hormonal secretions diminish with age. The best and simplest way to remove them is by electrodesiccation or snipping them off with surgical scissors; both cause little pain, mininal bleeding, and no scarring if done correctly. The treated areas may be a bit tender for a while, but if you avoid harsh scrubbing and eye makeup, you should be better than new in a few days.

Another mark of age is multiple skin-colored lesions called sebaceous adenomas. They appear on the face and cheeks and can be identified by a yellowish color and slight dimpling. Either electrodesiccation or trichloracetic acid will remove them.

Seborrheic keratoses—waxy, superficial growths that are yellowish, brown, or black, and of all possible shapes and sizes—can be dispatched with electrodesiccation, freezing, chemical peeling, or curettage (surgical scraping).

With so many possible ways of treating older skin, it is best to seek out a physician who performs a variety of procedures rather than someone who favors one alternative or another simply because he specializes in or knows how to do it best. Sometimes only combinatons of approaches are most effective—for example, a dermabrasion followed up with collagen and punch grafts. Avoid a doctor who recommends the same technique for just about all age-related problems.

Convinced that the leathery, lackluster look of aging skin is caused by a slowdown in the rate of cell renewal, researchers at the Clinic for Aging Skin in Philadelphia have devised a new topical form of rejuvenation. It is called **vitamin A** or **retinoic acid**, the prescription drug that has worked such wonders for acne (see Chapter 5). When dabbed on in a thin film, it accelerates the shedding of outermost cells and their replacement with newer ones from beneath to give skin a fresher, more youthful appearance. This natural peeling agent is also believed to stimulate collagen and blood vessel formation in the dermis (deeper layer), actually strengthening the supporting structures of the skin and keeping it better-toned and more resilient.

For reasons not yet known, vitamin A acid also appears to have a normalizing effect on damaged, irregular aging cells. After treatment, the surface layers look whole and healthy again, resembling those of younger skin. Mottling and liver spots are also reduced, since the more quickly shed cells have less time to soak up pigment from the lower layers.

Vitamin A acid therapy is considered especially valuable as a preventive treatment, keeping skin smooth and supple and eradicating fine creases before too many signs of aging have appeared. It may also help ward off local, potentially malignant growths called actinic keratoses, another consequence of prematurely seasoned skin.

Unless carefully supervised, this treatment can irritate and severely dry the skin. Fortunately, vitamin A acid (marketed as Retin-A) is available in a variety of strengths and bases to accommodate different skin types. So far, however, this topical drug has been officially approved only for acne. Its use on aging skin by the Philadelphia Clinic is still strictly experimental.

If your face is not overly dry, sensitive, or plagued with acne, you can help speed cell turnover yourself through a process called **epidermabrasion**. With a rough-textured washcloth, pumice stone, loofah, Buf-Puf, or with oatmeal grains, you can strip away the spent, flaky outer cells to make way for newer, younger layers from beneath. Some cosmetic researchers believe that such constant stimulation actually accelerates the rate at which cells migrate upward through layers of skin. By so doing, this technique may allow the cells to reach the top in better shape: more moist and supple, closer to their newborn state. While this still awaits proof, any invigorating facial workout will at least enhance circulation, giving your face a more glowing, fresh-scrubbed look.

Some skin care salons offer to erase your wrinkles via **electrolysis**. The electric needle is placed at an angle beneath a shallow fold or wrinkle. The immediate results are swelling, some irritation, and minor scaling, all of which camouflage the defect temporarily. But the skin reverts to its original look after the local injury heals, generally within several days. And the procedure is not without risk. Mottling and scarring are possible if the jolt of electricity is too powerful or carelessly applied.

A safer, vastly cheaper, and far more convenient alternative is to smooth beaten egg white into superficial cracks and creases with a fine-bristled brush. After it dries, apply foundation and other makeup as usual. This will temporarily tighten skin and glaze over any flaws, concealing them well for at least a few hours.

Another new approach to wrinkles is based on an ancient and revered oriental practice. **Acupuncture** is founded on the notion that the body's own natural tranquilizing and pain-relieving substances can be stimulated by applying pressure to certain major points, or meridians. Inserting needles into specific areas can relax key facial muscles and accelerate circulation. The effect is to ease superficial wrinkles and folds caused by these muscles being habitually tensed or contracted.

Proponents claim that acupuncture also helps contract

other key facial muscles, thereby improving tone and support for skin. Stepping up circulation may deliver more moisture to outer layers, helping to reduce the dryness responsible for fine surface lines. Since acupuncture reportedly relieves some internal conditions—which can show up as unflattering changes in color and complexion, blemishes, and other warnings—it may also indirectly improve the state of your skin.

About eight to fifteen tiny needles are painlessly implanted in the face, neck, calves, and hands to achieve the desired outcome. According to some claims, the effects may last up to two years, with periodic boosters required thereafter to maintain results. While American physicians and scientists remain skeptical about this newest application of an otherwise valid therapy, it is true that any method that reduces anxiety, whether hypnosis or meditation or acupuncture, will cause muscles to relax. So lines etched by facial tensions may well diminish as a result.

A handful of doctors (in Miami and elsewhere) have recently reported some moderate success with a newfangled technique, which has been called **biostimulation**. Directing their "cold" laser (instead of an acupuncture needle) at certain reflex points of the neck and face, they claim to tone, energize, and relax the skin and underlying tissues. After a series of twelve virtually painless treatments over a four- to six-week period, patients supposedly have noticeably fewer facial wrinkles and enjoy a rosier and more youthful complexion, because tapping the key reflex areas releases healthful energies, enhances circulation, and reduces the tensions that were contributing to facial lines and creases.

This method is not intended for severely damaged skin and does not completely smooth the face. Booster treatments are also called for every several months to maintain results.

Instead of cutting through or destroying tissue like the "hot" lasers used in surgery (which remove unsightly birthmarks, moles, and other stubborn blemishes), the "cold," far less intense cosmetic laser is reported to stimulate the production of collagen and elastin, two key supporting proteins, by causing a reaction in the cells' DNA and RNA, or genetic blueprint. This helps regenerate muscle fibers and improve facial tone, proponents claim. It also steps up circulation, which can itself enhance appearance.

The "cold" laser is being used experimentally in place of acupuncture needles at the same traditional points to relax and revitalize skin and achieve yet another nonsurgical lift. A deeply calming procedure, it may simply help iron out the superficial wrinkles and so-called worry lines caused by frequent frowning. The "cold" laser has been approved as a substitute for acupuncture, but the Food and Drug Administration is currently investigating its role in rejuvenating faces.

While this latest answer sounds promising to anyone seeking to erase a few years, always proceed with caution. Wait until a treatment or theory has been reliably tested before investing any time or money.

Nutritional Links

To look and stay youthful, skin must be nourished from within. That means eating mindfully—taking care to consume plenty of fresh foods as close to their natural state as possible.

Some scientists believe that the rate of cross-linking in skin, whereby tissues lose elasticity and moisture with age, can be slowed down by eating foods rich in natural protective nutrients called "antioxidants": These include vitamins A, C, E, the B-complex, especially B_1, B_5 and B_6, the minerals zinc and selenium, the amino acid cysteine (found in eggs and also available in tablet form), and citrus bioflavonoids (found in fruits and necessary for the absorption of vitamin C). That means a diet emphasizing fresh fruits and vegetables (sources of vitamins A and C), whole grains (for B-complex, E, selenium, and fiber) and a reduced intake of animal proteins, fats, and oils. Both saturated and unsaturated fats and oils may break down into highly destructive molecules called free radicals which are believed to accelerate the aging/cross-linking process in skin and other major organs.

Arguing that diet alone does not provide an adequate supply of antioxidants, some scientists advise taking supplements of these for added insurance. (Always check with a physician or nutrition professional before making any significant changes in your diet or vitamin-mineral intake.)

Damaged collagen *can* actually repair and replace itself, but this is a very slow process. Help retard and possibly reverse aging damage by protecting yourself from further sun exposure, living sensibly, and making sure you are well-supplied nutritionally. This will allow time for your body's natural healing processes to take effect. For complete guidelines on how to feed your skin, refer to Chapter 11.

Anti-Aging Cosmetics

A number of cosmetics companies have developed special products to combat wrinkles and other undesirables. How well do these work? As already mentioned, moisturizers can temporarily improve or mask the appearance of aging skin by filling in the outer layers with enough fluid to minimize fine lines. Many anti-wrinkle creams also contain an irritant to induce a slight swelling and yield the same short-term result.

The goal of many so-called youth-restoring treatment lines is primarily to restore to skin vital ingredients, such as oxygen and fluids, that are depleted with age, and also to reactivate the skin's natural functions, including swift cell turnover, moisture retention, and resistance to pollution.

Some formulas contain two kinds of oils: those with droplets small enough to penetrate the superficial layers of skin and those that are large enough to remain on the outside and create an external film. Proteins, for example, are big molecules, which form such a moisture-preserving barrier or screen. But despite claims, protein-based formulas are no more effective than such ordinary, basic oils as lanolin, petrolatum, mineral oil, and urea.

Certain raw materials in some products resemble the fatty components of skin that are responsible for keeping cells whole and rounded and the surface smooth and elastic. It is often claimed that they penetrate the deeper layers of the epidermis and provide a nourishing, oxygen-rich environment in which newly formed cells can develop and grow. These ingredients are often mingled with other so-called rejuvenators, typically one or more of the varieties of protein—collagen, elastin, amino acids, placenta, or hydrolyzed protein, for example—along with certain vitamins or minerals intended to preserve and protect these base-layer cells.

Unfortunately there is no evidence that collagen or any of its chemical cousins from a jar can affect or supplement the skin's own living tissue. No externally applied agent, however natural or native to real skin, can do anything to restore or reactivate a single cell. Results are at best fleeting and Cinderella-like, not worth the steep price tags boasted by such formulas. True, the water-retaining properties of the ingredients cause dried cells to fill out and wrinkles to flatten—but the magic will vanish by midnight. And while oily barriers can enhance moisture retention and resistance to the elements, there is no need to invest more than a few dollars to achieve such protection.

Certain abrasive cleansers designed for older skin exfoliate (slough away) the surface and stimulate sluggish cell renewal, but as yet there is no proof that regular use prods the skin to churn out new cells any faster than usual. And even if it does, a grainy washcloth will serve just as well. Remember, high cost, artful packaging, and inflated promises are not guarantees of a superior product.

Aside from corrective surgical procedures, minimizing sun exposure and staying healthy, well rested, and well nourished are the only "permanent" ways to combat the stigmata of aging skin.

Thus, the very best insurance against lined, leathery looks is sensible daily care, both outside and in. Cleanse and apply makeup with products suited to your skin type and with the gentlest possible hand. And become fanatical about ultraviolet rays. That means applying a sunscreen every day for the rest of your life. (Sunlight will penetrate your skin anyway, but a sunscreen will greatly soften the impact.) And do not just cover your face; remember the neck, chest, and back of hands, where age can leave an equally telling mark. A good pair of dark-tinted lenses will help prevent the crow's feet caused by squinting on overbright days and preserve the fragile skin around the eyes.

Not one of these safeguards requires more than simple planning or a few extra steps in your everyday routine. Such an easy investment is certainly well worth the dividend to come: your face at its best ten, twenty, even fifty years from now—a guaranteed lifetime of great-looking skin.

CHAPTER 9

BEFORE MAKEUP: STRAIGHT TALK ABOUT CLEAN SKIN

Everybody knows that skin needs regular cleansing, but not everyone understands why. Simply, proper cleansing sloughs away the topmost layer of old, dead skin cells, resulting in skin that looks brighter and feels fresher immediately.

If dead cells are not removed frequently and regularly, your complexion will tend to take on a dull, drab appearance. These cells begin to act like a veil, partially hiding the younger, vital, still-functioning skin underneath. In addition, if enough of the discarded, dehydrated cells are allowed to accumulate on the skin's surface, they can clog pores, causing a backup of secretions in the oil glands that can eventually lead to the formation of whiteheads, blackheads, and pimples.

Proper cleansing also eliminates other potential troublemakers, such as environmental grime and pollution, perspiration buildup, and any lingering accumulation of stale oils—both the natural kind, secreted by your skin's own oil glands, and the oil base of cosmetics.

Proper cleansing stimulates circulation, bringing an increased blood supply to all layers of the skin, creating a rosy glow on the surface, and nourishing the lower strata where new cells are continually being formed. The richer blood flow to lower layers encourages the growth of healthy new cells, which eventually make their way to the surface.

Proper cleansing does all this without unduly irritating the skin and robbing it of much-needed moisture.

In short, proper cleansing is important not only because it makes an immediate difference to the way your complexion looks and feels—glowing, fresher, softer—but also because each time you cleanse properly, you are investing in beauty insurance for the future.

Notice the emphasis on the phrase "proper cleansing." There are dozens of different ways to clean your face. But only a few of them—or possible only one method—will be right, or proper, for you.

For many women, discovering the way to clean skin is largely a matter of guesswork. Even some of the most sophisticated health- and beauty-conscious patients are confused about which products and methods to use. In fact, one of the most common questions asked of a dermatologist is: "What's the best way to clean my face?"

This is no surprise, since the array of different kinds (not to mention brands) of cleansing products on the market now is truly boggling. Instead of simplifying the matter, the advice offered in some of the popular beauty books is often conflicting (and sometimes downright erroneous), and only adds to the confusion.

What's more, almost everyone has some well-meaning friend or relative who swears that her own radiant, clear complexion is the result of religiously using a particular brand of cleansing cream morning and night or of scrubbing vigorously with a certain exotic soap.

The truth is, Cream X or Soap Y may indeed add to the marvelous good looks of someone you know. But it is always a mistake to assume that the cleansing products and methods used by a famous television personality, or even by your own sister, will work wonders for you, too. The cleansing routine that is just right for one woman may be the worst possible choice for another.

For example, an oily-skinned patient decided to follow a cleansing regime that seemed to be working well for an oily-skinned friend of hers. The routine involved scrubbing three times a day with cleansing granules, each scrubbing followed by an application of a strong medicated de-greasing lotion. After less than a week, her skin was so reddened and sore that she could hardly bear to touch it. What went wrong? Though she knew she had an oily complexion, like her friend, she did not realize that her own skin was also quite sensitive and could not take such harsh treatment.

Another patient, whose skin was basically normal, read a beauty book that discouraged the use of soaps of any kind. So this woman switched to cleansing with a heavy cream and soon began to have problems with minor blemishes and blackheads. The point of this little story is not that cream cleansing is bad (it can be excellent for certain kinds of skin), but that this particular woman had chosen the wrong type of product for her skin and neglected to follow the cleansing with an astringent or other product to remove the cream, grime, and dead cell debris.

The point is simply this: No matter what miracles are promised on the labels of those glamorously packaged tubes, bottles, and bars of cleansing products, no matter how the most fascinating woman you know cleans her face, no matter what the beauty books tell you, the deciding factor with regard to the best way of treating your complexion is your own individual skin type.

Roundup: Cleansing Products

If you have read Chapter 2, you already know your skin profile. If you skipped that chapter, go back and read it now. In the pages that follow we will be prescribing proper cleansing products and techniques for each of the various skin types.

YOUR SKIN

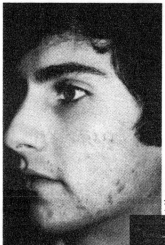

Acne before treatment with Retin-A and benzoyl peroxide

Micera

Acne after treatment with Retin-A and benzoyl peroxide

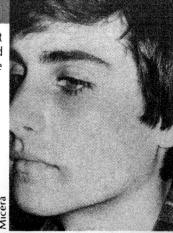

Micera

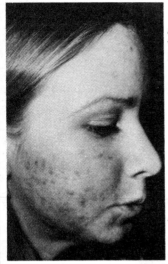

Acne before treatment
with Retin-A and
benzoyl peroxide

S. Merchant

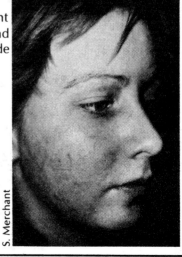

Acne after treatment
with Retin-A and
benzoyl peroxide

S. Merchant

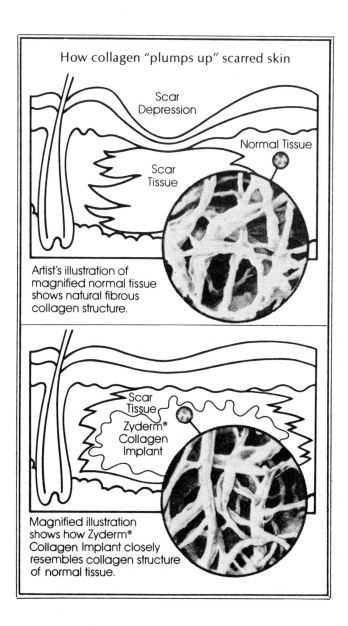

How collagen "plumps up" scarred skin

Scar Depression

Normal Tissue

Scar Tissue

Artist's illustration of magnified normal tissue shows natural fibrous collagen structure.

Scar Tissue

Zyderm® Collagen Implant

Magnified illustration shows how Zyderm® Collagen Implant closely resembles collagen structure of normal tissue.

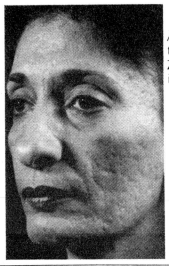

Acne scars before
treatment with
Zyderm® Collagen
implant

Acne scars after
treatment with
Zyderm® Collagen
implant

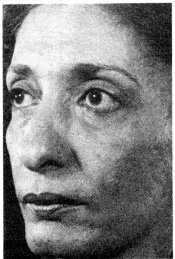

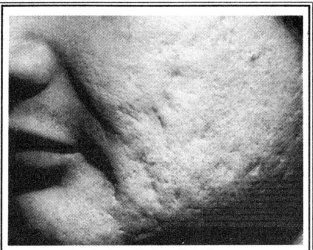

Acne scarring before Zyderm® Collagen treatment

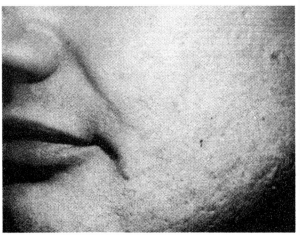

Acne scarring after Zyderm® Collagen treatment

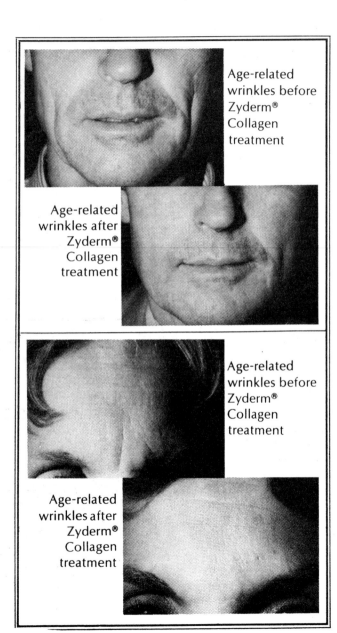

Age-related wrinkles before Zyderm® Collagen treatment

Age-related wrinkles after Zyderm® Collagen treatment

Age-related wrinkles before Zyderm® Collagen treatment

Age-related wrinkles after Zyderm® Collagen treatment

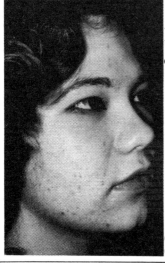

Acne scars before treatment with chemical peeling

E. Cser

Acne scars after treatment with chemical peeling

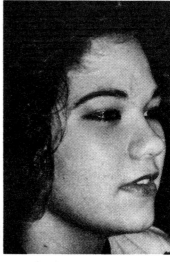

E. Cser

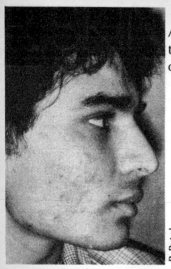

Acne scars before treatment with dermabrasion

P. Patel

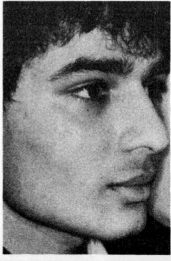

Acne scars after treatment with dermabrasion

P. Patel

But first it is important to get a little more acquainted with the cleansing products themselves, because the best patient (and readers), those who show the most dramatic improvement, are always those who are best informed.

Soaps

The oldest cleansing product of all (plain water except-ed), soap is made by mixing an alkali with a natural fat and water. Other cleansing products that we tend to think of as soap—because they look, feel, and smell like soap, and often come in rectangular or oval-shaped bar form—are made with synthetic compounds and are more properly called detergents.

Don't let the word "detergent" turn you off. Cosmetic chemists can and do manipulate detergent formulas in hundreds of different ways. Some are gentler than the mildest toilet soaps. Others have special grease-cutting properties that some true soaps lack. Also, in hard water areas of the country, a detergent cleanser is often easier to rinse off and tends to leave less residue on the skin.

Obviously, all soaps and their detergent counterparts are not alike. Some are too harsh for certain skin types, while others may be too gentle for maximum results. A few soaps and detergents contain ingredients that can lead to problems for still other types.

Though soaps definitely fall into the toiletry category, many are exempt from Federal Food and Drug Administra-tion labeling laws that require labels on cosmetics to carry a list of ingredients. The exceptions are detergent cleans-ers and those products (antibacterial soaps, for example) that claim to do more than simply get skin clean.

But the special properties—good and bad—of soaps and detergents need not remain a mystery just because ingredients are not always listed on the wrapper. You can tell a lot about a soap or detergent from its name or the way it is described on the wrapper; this will usually indi-cate which of the following categories it belongs to.

Baby soaps: Formulated to cleanse tender young skin gently, baby soaps are mild products often well suited to normal and moderately dry skin. Many sensitive skin types can tolerate a good baby soap better than ordinary toilet bars.

Castile soaps: The principle fatty ingredient of these soaps is olive oil, rather than the tallow, hydrogenated vegetable oil, and sometimes even garbage greases used in many other soaps. It may be because olive oil is more appealing than tallow and garbage grease that castile soaps have won a reputation for their purity and mildness. However, these soaps confer no special benefits on the skin. They are simply good middle-of-the-road cleansers, neither especially rich nor especially drying.

Cocoa butter soaps: Cocoa butter sounds delicious, but that is never the point where skin cleansers (or any skin products) are concerned. In these soaps, cocoa butter replaces the tallow and vegetable oil used as the fatty ingredient in many other soaps. Some if not all cocoa butter soaps belong in the Superfatted category (see below). One important point to keep in mind about these soaps is that they may cause allergic reactions, especially in those who are allergic to chocolate.

Detergent soaps: As mentioned earlier, detergent cleansers are not necessarily any more harsh than soaps made with natural ingredients. In fact, some are very gentle but at the same time have great de-oiling properties.

In one recent study, a detergent bar (Dove) was found to be less irritating and produced less scaling of the skin than any of the eighteen other popular cleansers tested. Yet Dove, if used with very warm water, is a great de-oiler. This is not meant to tout Dove above all other cleansers, but merely to stress the point that detergents are excellent products for certain skin types and under certain circumstances.

How can you tell if the soap you are buying is a detergent? For one thing, a detergent cleanser must have its ingredients listed on label or wrapper; among those may be names that include the terms "sulfate" or "sulfonate." (To complicate matters somewhat, some true soaps also have ingredient listings, even though they are not required to do so. However, if "natural fat," "tallow," or "coconut oil" is mentioned on the label or wrapper, chances are the product is not a detergent.)

Deodorant soaps: These have as ingredients chemicals formulated to kill bacteria that live on secretions from the apocrine glands (a type of sweat-producing gland). If these bacteria are allowed to thrive, unpleasant body odor may be the result. Deodorant soaps may be helpful in controlling these, though for most people frequent bathing with any soap is as effective. Avoid using a deodorant soap as a facial cleanser. There are no apocrine glands on the face, and there is still some question about minor side effects of the antibacterial agents in these soaps. Since facial skin may be more easily irritated, and is certainly more visible than skin on the rest of the body, there is no reason for you to use a deodorant soap with questionable ingredients when there are so many alternatives to choose from.

Floating soaps: Ivory is the prime example, a good all-around toilet soap, gentle and neither overly drying nor very rich. It floats because of the air trapped inside it and because of the unusually high percentage of water in its formulation.

French-milled soaps: These have a lower alkaline content than many other soaps, which means they tend to be less drying to the skin. If dry skin is your problem, you need not assume, however, that nothing but a good French milled soap is fit to use on your complexion. These soaps do have a silky, luxurious texture, but they carry an equally luxurious price tag. Many detergent soaps, such as Dove, Caress, and Purpose, are just as low in alkalinity and cost considerably less.

Fruit, vegetable, and herbal soaps: Though we do not have sales figures to prove it, these soaps must be very popular now, since they are on display in pharmacies, department stores, health food stores, dime and novelty stores, and even souvenir shops along the highways. Presumably their popularity has to do with the association people naturally make between fresh, wholesome, unblemished vegetables and fruits and the way we would all like our skin to look. Far from being the wholesome all-natural products many people take them to be, fruit, vegetable, and herbal soaps may actually contain more drying alcohol and chemical preservatives—put there to stabilize the fruit, vegetable, or herbal extracts—than many ordinary toilet soaps. That yummy fruity scent is probably a blending of dozens of fragrance chemicals; no natural scent could withstand the soap manufacturing process. As for the color, it is probably dye.

Medicated soaps: Also known as antimicrobial and bacteriostatic cleansers, these contain antibacterial ingredients for the purpose of controlling or killing skin bacteria. They are not ordinarily recommended for any but acne-ridden skin.

Milled soaps: Most ordinary toilet soaps fall into this category. Milling is the manufacturing process by which soap chips or pellets are squeezed and kneaded and finally made into bars. These soaps contain perfume and coloring (as do almost all soaps), as well as varying amounts of fatty acids and alkalies. Their cost is modest; most do a good job of getting skin clean, and, used with discretion, they are an appropriate choice for many normal, oily, and combination skins. (Incidentally, French-milled soap is in fact multi-milled. Ivory, on the other hand, undergoes no milling process.)

Sulfur soaps: Sulfur is an ingredient in many soaps used for the treatment of acne. One special property of sulfur is that it tends to slow the skin's oil production. It is also a mild peeling agent, which means that a sulfur soap will remove more of the topmost layer of dead skin cells than most others. When a soap contains sulfur, the fact will be mentioned on the wrapper.

Superfatted soaps: As you might guess, superfatted soaps have extra amounts of fatty substances—usually coconut oil, cocoa butter, cold cream, or lanolin—added during the manufacturing process. This makes them a good choice for many (but not all) people with dry skin. Some of these soaps do a less than thorough job of dissolving and removing facial oils. In fact, one of the properties of some superfatted soaps is a tendency to leave a thin film of oil on the skin, which remains even after thorough rinsing. (This can be either good or bad, depending on your skin type.) Other superfatted soaps rinse off very nicely.

Transparent soaps: If you have ever used one, you may have been delighted with the silken texture of your skin immediately after rinsing. Neutrogena, the largest manufacturer of transparent soaps, now churns out five variations: regular, non-scented; regular, scented; dry skin formula; acne (or oily skin) formula; one especially for babies. All are mild, gentle cleaners with low-alkaline formulations.

One caution: These products cost more than ordinary toilet soaps and have a tendency to melt down to a mere sliver if kept in a wet soap dish. Transparent soap will last longer if covered with plastic wrap after each use.

Creams, Cream-Type, and Lotion Cleansers

Some creamy and lotion cleansers are actually liquefied versions of soaps or detergents. We will pass over these for now and concentrate instead on conventional cold creams, cleansing creams, and their lotion variations.

Though many creams and lotions do an exceptional job of dissolving makeup—better and quicker than soaps and detergents in many instances—traditional creams and lotions just do not lift away enough of the top layer of old dead skin cells to make much difference. Except for those rare individuals who simply cannot tolerate soap or detergent cleansers, these products are not the best ways to good, basic, all-around skin care.

Unless you wash with soap and water after tissuing off the cream, a film invariably remains on the skin. Since many creams also contain both alcohol and soap or soaplike substances, both dehydrating agents, even a very oily cream cleanser may eventually have a drying effect if not thoroughly and completely rinsed away.

Cleansing creams: If you think you are avoiding soap by using a cleansing cream instead of washing your face, you may be mistaken. As mentioned previously, some cleansing creams contain soap or soaplike ingredients. Typical ones also contain mineral oil, wax, alcohol, preservatives, and something to make them smell good.

These creams are meant to be applied to the skin, then wiped off with a tissue. According to the ad writers for these products, when the cream is removed, so is every last trace of grime, old makeup, stale oil, and other soil. Well, some of that stuff comes off, but every last trace? Hardly. Cleansing creams simply do not clean as effectively as soap and water.

Cleansing lotions: Most of these are very similar in their chemical makeup to cleansing creams, the primary difference being that additional water in the formulation gives them a thick, liquid consistency.

Liquefying cleansing creams: These are still another variation on the basic cleansing cream. Ingredients are typical, except that they have been formulated to melt—liquefy—at body temperature. Albolene cream, a very gentle mineral-oil based liquefying cream, is an especially quick and efficient makeup remover, safe enough even for cleaning away eye makeup.

Cold cream: The typical cold cream has a somewhat simpler formula than a cleansing cream, being mainly water, mineral oil, wax (often beeswax), borax or some other alkaline ingredient that has a softening effect on the skin, preservatives, and perfume. Like cleansing creams and lotions, cold creams are applied to the face, then wiped off. In the process, most but not all dirt and makeup are removed. Because the typical cold cream contains little or no alcohol, the film left behind after it has been tissued off may not be as drying as cleansing cream residue.

Milky cleansers: Sometimes called cleansing milks, these are usually whitish in color but ordinarily contain not a drop of the dairy product for which they are named. Instead, ingredients are likely to include soap or soaplike substances, water, alcohol, and mineral oil. So much soap is found in these cleansers that some experts in cosmetics chemistry insist that these products are really liquid soaps.

Washable creams: These are also called rinsing creams. The distinguishing characteristic of these products, which are basically cleansing creams (sometimes a little camphor or menthol is added for an extra tingle), is that they can be rinsed off with water. Washable creams do a pretty good job of dissolving and removing makeup and grime and are better at lifting away dead skin cells than many other cream-type products. But they are not as good as most soaps and detergents.

The trouble with this kind of cream is that the user may feel she is getting the best of both worlds—the gentleness of a cream combined with the effectiveness of a soap—since, after all, like soap, the product is rinsed away with a few splashes from the tap. Unfortunately, clogged pores and eventually blemishes are too often the result when people with normal-to-oily skin rely solely on washing creams for cleansing.

Granules and Scrubs

A third category of cleanser is composed of products variously designated "cleansing grains," "granular soaps," "granular foams," "scrubbing grains," and "facial scrubs." Some come in powder form and are meant to be moistened and applied to the face with water; others come in bar form; still others are soaplike foams. Quite a few contain sulfur or other drying agents.

What they all have in common is the inclusion in their makeup of tiny grains, often of pumice of polyethelene. When briskly scrubbed into the skin, these granular products not only cleanse but also abrade away the topmost layer of dead skin cells—and then some. This abrasive action is called sloughing or exfoliating.

Many patients find that vigorous massaging with a granular cleanser helps control oil and even removes blackheads. They also like the pink glow it brings to their complexion temporarily.

These products should rarely be used on a daily basis, and never on a sensitive skin. When they are used too often and too enthusiastically, skin tends to become tender and irritated.

Follow-Up Treatments

The products we are concerned with in this section are known variously as astringents, fresheners, clarifying lotions, toners, refining lotions, pore lotions, and . . . the list could go on and on.

There is a lot of overlapping among these products. One company's clarifying lotion may be very similar to another company's toner or refining lotion or astringent. Because of the overlap, it is next to impossible to divide products in this group into meaningful categories.

However, some form of follow-up treatment is advisable. These liquids and lotions are all formulated to remove any traces of cleanser that rinsing or tissuing has left behind. They also make the skin look and feel fresher, smoother, and tighter, which is a pleasant, bracing way to finish up any cleansing routine.

In addition, some of these products contain ingredients that puff up skin tissue temporarily, making pores seem to disappear—at least for a while. Others have pronounced sloughing or exfoliating properties or promote a pleasant rosy glow. Still others act in several of the above ways at once and contain moisturizing ingredients as well.

There are a few important things to keep in mind when selecting a follow-up treatment.

Read labels carefully to make sure of what you are getting. If you want an exfoliating product that will peel away dead skin cells, look for one that mentions sloughing or exfoliation on the label.

Keep in mind that the more alcohol in a product, the more drying it will tend to be. Lists of ingredients on toiletries labels are like those on food labels. The first-mentioned ingredient is the one present in the product in greatest quantity. If you want a drying product, look for one that lists alcohol first on the label. If you want to avoid dryness, try to find a product that lists alcohol in second or third place and that also contains moisturizing ingredients such as glycerin and allantoin.

Remember that most companies make several versions of the same treatment product, modifying them to suit different skin types. The skin type for which the product is deemed most appropriate will be prominently indicated on the label: dry, normal, oily, and in some cases combination and sensitive. Obviously, start with the one that is typed for your skin. (If you have combination skin, but the product in question does not come in a version to match, choose the "normal" version.)

If the product seems too harsh, try using it every other day for a while instead of daily. Skin is adaptable and sometimes learns to tolerate certain products in this way. If the product still seems too harsh, backtrack a notch. In other words, if you bought a treatment recommended for normal skin, switch to the dry skin version and see what happens.

Face-Cleansing Basics

Here is some basic cleansing advice that applies to all skin types.

Before cleansing, pin or tie hair back securely from your face. Otherwise, you might be tempted to skimp on cleansing—or avoid entirely—the all-important areas along the hairline.

Though technically your face ends at the jawbone, do not stop cleansing there. Apply soap or cream cleanser well down onto the neckline so that every bit of makeup is removed. Remember, though, that neck skin is particularly sensitive, so do not use cleansing grains or follow-up products on your neck.

Be as gentle as possible when applying soap or cream cleansers. Vigorous massaging will not make the product work any more effectively, and the less you pull and stretch at your face the better it is for your skin in the long run.

Do not overdo cleansing. Twice a day—once in the morning and once at bedtime—is enough for most people. If you are going directly from office to party of theater and want to freshen your makeup beforehand, remove the old makeup quickly with an oil-based lotion, astringent-saturated pad, or even a Wash N'Dry. Your skin may not be spanking clean after this quick cleanup, but the alternative—a third full-scale cleansing—just is not necessary under the circumstances and may in fact be more than your skin can comfortably tolerate.

You should be able to get your regular morning and evening cleansing routines over and done with in two minutes or less. If you are spending much more time than that on cleansing your skin, you are probably overdoing it, and your complexion may suffer as a result.

Do not underestimate the importance of rinsing off soap or detergent-type cleansers. Your goal is to remove as much as possible. Rinsing cannot be stressed too much, so aim for about fifteen splashes with running water. (Never fill the bathroom basin and rinse over and over again with the same dirty water.) Start with tepid water and gradually adjust the temperature so that the final few rinses are icy cold.

Be flexible and use common sense. In the next section, different products and procedures will be prescribed for different skin types. These recommendations are based on years of training and clinical practice, and have helped many patients to better, sometimes beautiful, complexions, and can probably do the same for you. However, without a dermatologist's regular care you have to be the final judge of whether the products and techniques suggested here are actually benefiting your skin.

In other words, give those products and techniques a chance, do not be inflexible about modifying them if common sense and your mirror dictate a change.

Cleansing Prescriptions for
Dry Skin

Dry Skin—Young
Although young dry skin gives more leeway than mature dry skin, gentle treatment is important.

Morning Cleansing: Assuming you went to bed with a freshly washed face, start off in the morning by cleansing with a mild toilet soap (for instance, Ivory), a baby soap, or a superfatted soap or detergent such as Basis, Dove, or Clinique's Soap Mild. Deodorant soaps and soaps with pronounced fragrance are not for you.

To wash, wet your face thoroughly with tepid—not hot—water, lather up and apply the cleanser. One application is enough. Fingertip application is best.

But what if you prefer a washcloth? The best advice is to learn to prefer your fingertips. A washcloth is too abrasive for dry skin and may aggravate your problems. However, if a washcloth is a lifelong habit you can't seem to break, then use it, but skip the follow-up treatment. An abrasive washcloth plus toner or astringent may be more than your skin can tolerate.

Rinse well, starting with tepid water, gradually adjusting the temperature to cold.

Pat dry with a soft, fluffy towel. No hard rubbing.

Apply astringent, toner, or other follow-up product formulated for dry skin.

Evening Cleansing: Same as for morning, except that your

first step should be to remove makeup with an oil-base cream or lotion. Do not forget that there are special removers for eye makeup.

Dry Skin—Mature
Mature dry skin tends to be dryer and may be somewhat more sensitive than young dry skin. *Supergentle* is the key word.

Morning Cleansing: Wash with a mild, unscented toilet soap or baby soap, or a superfatted soap, if your skin can tolerate it. Lather once and apply with your fingertips.

If you do not like soap, or if you find it too drying, try a soapless cleanser. One particularly good for mature dry skin is Keri Facial Cleanser, a gentle product with added moisturizers.

Rinse well, starting with tepid water, gradually adjusting the temperature to cold.

Pat dry gently with a soft towel. If your skin is very dry and on the sensitive side, you might find blow-drying more soothing than blotting with a towel. You will need a hair dryer for this. Set the appliance on warm, hold it in one hand at least six inches from your face. With the other hand gently rub away excess moisture. As drying proceeds, reset appliance to the cool setting.

If your skin can tolerate it, apply a gentle toner or astringent formulated for dry skin. (Look for the kind that mentions moisturizing ingredients on the label.)

Evening Cleansing: Same as for morning cleansing, unless you have been wearing makeup all day. If that is the case, start out by removing makeup with an oil-base cream or lotion. Incidentally, the Keri Facial Cleanser mentioned above is a good makeup remover also. You need not use it twice in one session (once to remove makeup and once to cleanse); a single application will suffice.

Dry Skin—Sensitive
Of all skin types, yours is the most delicate. The cleansing products you use should be the mildest, most gentle available. Otherwise, as a general rule, the less you do to and for your skin, the better.

Morning Cleansing: Wash with a mild soapless product such as Lowila. (If your skin is sensitive all over, you can also use Lowila in the tub and as a shampoo.) Other products recommended for dry sensitive skin are Oilatum and Clinique Cleansing Cream Subtype 1 (the latter is also an excellent makeup remover).

If itching occurs, you might want to try one of the following: Alpha Keri, Lubath, Mapo, Nutraspa, Aveeno, Domol, Balnetar, Kauma. Use according to label instructions.

Obviously, if you have chosen a cleansing cream, you will not need to rinse; simply remove the cream with light dabbing motions.

Soap and soap-type products should be thoroughly rinsed with tepid running water. Finish with cool water.

Blot dry with a fluffy towel. (Important: Be aware that the residue of chemicals used in certain fabric softeners may be irritating to your sensitive skin.) Or blow your face dry, using the method suggested for mature dry skin. Be sure to hold the blower at least six inches from your face, and take your time. You want to blow your skin perfectly dry. (This method takes a little longer, but if you can spend the extra minutes, do so; blow-drying is gentler than towel-drying.)

If your skin is very sensitive, use no follow-up product. Remember, your type of skin does best when products and procedures are kept to a minimum.

Evening Cleansing: Same as morning cleansing, unless you wear makeup, in which case it should be removed with a very mild oil-base cream or lotion.

A few general tips for dry skin: If your skin is dry all over, quick warm showers are better than long hot soaks in the tub. Apply a mild nonscented emollient to the entire body immediately after leaving the shower.

Do not use granular scrubs or other abrasives on your face. However, assuming that the skin on the rest of your body is not extraordinarily sensitive, you can, if you like, smooth upper arms, elbows, knees, heels, etc., with abrasive products.

Moisture is enormously important in treating dry skin—both the moisture in your immediate environment and moisturizing products for your face and body. (See Chapter 2.)

Cleansing Prescriptions for Normal Skin

Normal Skin—Young
Normal skin, with its minimal problems and good balance between dryness and oiliness, at least sounds as though it would be easy to care for. Usually it is, especially normal young skin. But don't be too casual and take your normal skin for granted. It is easily nudged over the line toward dryness on the one hand or toward the problems associated with excess oil on the other.

Morning Cleansing: Of course you removed makeup before you went to bed last night, so the first step in morning cleansing is to wash your face. Use a mild toilet soap, such as Ivory or Camay. Other good choices are Neutragena Regular, Dove, and Basis. If your pocketbook can stand the strain, Clinique for normal skin is excellent.

To wash, wet your face thoroughly with tepid water (hot water tends to be drying), lather up and apply the cleanser with your fingertips. One rich application of lather is sufficient.

Rinse thoroughly, starting with tepid running water, gradually adjusting the temperature to cold.

Blot completely dry with a soft towel.

Do not regularly use a washcloth, buff puff, complexion brush, or other physical exfoliator, since these can remove protective natural oils all too well. And remember, it does not take much to swing normal skin over to the dry side.

However, if you must, use an exfoliator gently, occasionally (at most twice a week), and for only short periods of time. Whenever you do, chose a follow-up product labeled for normal skin and use it after each cleansing session.

Evening Cleansing: Same as for morning, except that you should use a creamy or oil-type lotion for quick makeup removal before washing.

Normal Skin—Mature

People in this skin-category often started out with oily skin, which became dryer—closer to normal—with passing time. However, after years of thinking about and treating their skin as oily, many women find it difficult to give up oily-skin cleansing techniques and learn to treat their complexion more gently. However, it is important that they do so; otherwise dry skin problems may result.

Morning Cleansing: Assuming makeup was removed the night before, start by washing with a mild soap. The cleansing products and techniques recommended for normal young skin would be appropriate.

An even gentler alternative would be a mild soapless cleanser such as Keri Facial Cleanser, which contains water, glycerine, and moisturizers. This product can also be used to remove makeup.

Cream cleansing is a third alternative for mature women with dry skin who just do not feel comfortable about using a soap or detergent for complexion cleansing. The best of the cream cleansers for mature dry skin are those based on the beeswax-borax system. (These ingredients will be listed on the product label; to make life simpler, ask a good pharmacist to recommend a cream made with beeswax and borax.)

Mature normal skin usually is too delicate for physical exfoliation with a washcloth, buff puff, or complexion brush. Cleansing granules and scrubs are also off limits.

If you want mild exfoliation, choose a follow-up product for normal skin that has a mention of exfoliating properties on the label. If redness, flakiness, or irritation occur, use the product every other day only or switch to one labeled for dry skin.

Evening Cleansing: Same as for morning cleansing except for makeup removal. If you are using the Keri Facial Cleanser for general cleansing, you can simplify your life by using it for makeup removal, too. The same applies to beeswax-borax cream cleansers.

Normal Skin—Sensitive
Yes, it is possible to have skin that is normal (not too dry, not too oily) and sensitive (easily irritated) at one and the same time. Not only is it possible, normal sensitive skin is a sub-type frequently seen by dermatologists.

Morning Cleansing: If your skin is just moderately sensitive, probably you can safely follow the basic cleansing routine prescribed for mature normal skin. Just use smaller amounts of the suggested products, apply them with a lighter touch, and perhaps shorten the time they are in contact with your skin.

Do not skimp on rinsing, however. Fifteen splashes, starting with tepid tap water, gradually adjusting temperature to cold, is still the rule.

Blot dry with a fluffy towel. (Be aware that the chemical residue of certain fabric softeners may cause problems for your sensitive skin.)

Or air-dry your face by holding a blower-type hair dryer set on warm at least six inches away from the skin. Gently rub off moisture with one hand while the other hand holds the dryer. Switch the appliance to the cool setting to finish drying. This method of drying skin after rinsing takes longer, but is gentler than towel-drying.

If your skin can tolerate a follow-up product, use a gentle freshener or astringent with added moisturizers. Even though your skin is normal, products labeled for sensitive or dry skin may give you best results.

Evening Cleansing: Same as for morning, except that makeup should be removed with a gentle cream or oil-based lotion.

If your skin is extremely sensitive, you may need to follow the ultragentle cleansing procedures described in the section on sensitive dry skin.

A few general tips for normal skin: Even though your skin is classified as normal, it probably has a very slight tendency to be either a bit dry or a bit oily. Seasonal changes may exaggerate the tendency. Winter may accentuate dryness while summer heat and humidity may bring on the oil. Adjust your cleansing routine accordingly, adapting some of the dry skin products and techniques to suit your needs when necessary and switching to oily skin products and techniques if skin begins to take on a greasy shine.

Unless you are going through an oily phase, do not use granular scrubs on facial skin. (When the oily stage has passed, discontinue the scrubs.) You can safely use abrasives to smooth other areas of your body, however, though you should avoid these products altogether if body skin is sensitive.

Cleansing Prescriptions for Combination Skin

While dry skin is usually associated with maturity and oily skin with youth, combination skin seems to occur about equally in all but the very oldest and youngest age groups.

When it comes to cleansing, combination skin presents a unique problem or two, because you are treating both relatively dry and relatively oily skin at once. (Some beauty books suggest buying two separate sets of products, one set to cleanse the oily T-zone, the other for the somewhat dryer cheek areas.)

Choose a follow-up treatment (astringent, toner, freshener, clarifying, or exfoliating lotion, etc.) recommended for combination skin. You may have trouble finding one, as many companies market products only for dry, normal, and oily skin. If you cannot find the treatment you want in combination skin formula, buy the version intended for normal skin. Use according to manufacturer's instructions, but apply it a bit more vigorously and allow it to remain longer on the T-zone area.

Combination Skin—Mature
In contrast to younger combination skin, mature combination complexions are often just slightly oily in the T-zone and relatively dry on cheeks and other areas. That is because of the natural tendency for oil production to slow as time goes on. However, even young women with minimal shine in the T-zone and greater dryness elsewhere can use the following techniques.

Morning Cleansing: If your morning face is makeup-free, start by washing with a mild soap or detergent bar. You can choose from among all the products recommended for young combination skin.

To wash, wet your face with tepid water, splashing slightly warmer water on the oily T-zone. Lather up and massage the cleanser first into the T-zone. Since your skin is only slightly oily in the T-zone, you do not need to cleanse that area too long or too vigorously. Without relathering, use your fingertips to cleanse the remainder of your face.

A washcloth, buff puff, loofah, or complexion brush should be used gently, if at all, and no more often than every other day.

Rinse thoroughly with running water. Start out with warm, not hot, water in the T-zone and gradually adjust the temperature to tepid for the rest of your face. Finish rinsing with cold water.

Blot dry with a fluffy towel.

Choose a follow-up treatment recommended for combination skin. If you cannot locate what you want in a combination formula, buy the normal skin version, and see how that works. Since your skin is mostly dry with only slight oiliness in the T-zone, you might find that a follow-up treatment in a dry skin formulation works even better for you.

Evening Cleansing: Same as for morning cleansing, except that makeup, including eye makeup, should be removed first with a mild cream or oil-base lotion.

Combination Skin—Sensitive
Morning Cleansing: If your skin is only slightly sensitive, follow the same basic cleansing routine prescribed for mature combination skin. You might get better results if you use smaller amounts of the products, apply them more gently, and allow them less time in contact with your skin.

Do not use a washcloth, buff puff, loofah, or complexion brush.

Rinse thoroughly, starting with tepid tap water, gradually adjusting temperature to cold.

Blot dry with a fluffy towel; be aware that certain fabric softeners may leave a residue that irritates sensitive skin.

Gentler but more time-consuming than towel-drying is drying your face with a blower-type hair dryer held at least six inches from your skin. Aim the dryer with one hand. Gently rub away moisture from skin with the other. Start drying with appliance on the warm setting. Finishing the job with on cool.

If your skin can tolerate a follow-up treatment, use a gentle astringent, toner, or clarifying lotion recommended for sensitive skin. If you cannot find one, experiment with mild products formulated for normal or dry skin.

If your skin is extremely sensitive, you may want to try the mild cleansing techniques described in the section on sensitive dry skin.

Evening Cleansing: Same as for morning cleansing.

A few general tips for combination skin: Cleansing combination skin can be tricky. Even if your T-zone is very oily, do not make the mistake of adopting some of the aggressive de-oiling techniques described next in this chapter. If you do, your dry skin areas may become even dryer and worse—tender, red, and irritated.

The one exception to the above rule is the occasional use of a granular cleanser or scrub applied to the T-zone only. Choose one of the gentler products in this category—a mild oatmeal scrub, for example—and use no more often than once or twice a week. This cleansing technique will help to reduce the shine in oily areas, making your skin seem more all of a kind.

Facial saunas, another of the aggressive oily skin treatments discussed in the next section, are not for you. Though steam-cleaning may reduce oiliness in the T-zone, it will also promote dryness elsewhere. The result, a dryer, more sensitive combination skin.

One way to counteract that annoying shine down the center of your face is to carry a packet of special oil-absorbent tissues with you everywhere and blot gently whenever the skin gets out of hand. These tissues are not for naked skin only. They are equally good at blotting up excess oil that seeps through makeup.

Cleansing Prescriptions for Oily Skin

Though oily skin and acne often go hand in hand, the cleansing techniques described in this section are for acne-free oily skin. (If acne is a problem, turn to Chapters 3, 4, and 5.)

Oily skin tends to be thicker and less sensitive than other skin types. This gives you more leeway with regard to using stronger products and more vigorous treatments.

Oily Skin—Young
Skin is usually oiliest during the teen years and early- to mid-twenties, and the aggressive routine that follows is designed to help correct and de-grease oil-gushing young skin. However, some older people whose skin continues to to excessively oily may also benefit from the routine.

Morning Cleansing: You can choose from a number of special de-oiling products to wash your makeup-free morning face. The most aggressive of all are the granular scrubs, which de-grease and exfoliate in one operation.

Products such as Pernox, Brasivol (which is available in three formulations: fine, medium, and coarse granules), and Komex (which is somewhat gentler, because the granules it contains dissolve rather quickly) all come to mind.

Use these products according to label instructions. When lathering is called for, use very warm, but not hot, tap water.

Do not use a washcloth, buff puff, loofah, complexion brush, or other physical exfoliator to apply products containing grains or granules.

Rinse thoroughly, starting with very warm tap water, adjusting temperature gradually to cold.

Blot dry with a soft towel.

Follow up with an astringent, toner, or clarifying lotion labeled for oily skin.

Evening Cleansing: Same as morning cleansing, except that the first step is to remove makeup and eye makeup. Since you probably wear water-based instead of oil-based makeup (and if you don't, you should), look for a cream or lotion designed to dissolve surface oil and water-based makeup.

Oily Skin—Mature

Many beauty books written by "experts" who are not usually dermatologists assume that once past the age of thirty-five or so, oily skin ceases to be a problem. However, almost every day dermatologists see people of thirty-five, forty, and up (way up), whose skin is still decidedly oily.

It is true, though, that oily mature skin tends to gush less than oily young skin, and the following cleansing routine takes this into account. (Younger readers whose skin is not excessively oily may also benefit from this routine.)

Morning Cleansing: Wash makeup-free skin with a degreasing but nongranular soap or cleanser such as Cuticura,

Clearasil Soap, or KeriKleen. Milder but still effective are toilet soaps such as Ivory and Neutragena for Oily skin and detergent bars such as Purpose and Basis.

To wash, wet your face thoroughly with very warm water, lather up and apply the cleanser, using your fingertips to work it gently over all skin surfaces. After rinsing thoroughly you may lather and apply the cleanser a second time.

An alternative to fingertip application is to use a physical exfoliator such as a washcloth, buff puff, loofah, or complexion brush.

Rinse thoroughly, starting with very warm water, gradually adjusting the temperature to cold.

Blot dry with a soft towel.

Follow up with an astringent, toner, or clarifying lotion labeled for oily skin. (Note: If you prefer to apply cleanser with a physical exfoliator, you may experience an unpleasant burning or stinging sensation when oily skin follow-up products are used on the skin. In that case you have several options. Use the physical exfoliator less often—say, every other day instead of daily—or stop using it entirely; switch to a milder follow-up product, perhaps one labeled for normal skin. However, do avoid follow-up products that contain moisturizers.)

Evening Cleansing: Same as for morning cleansing, but start off with a cream or lotion-type product designed to dissolve skin oils and remove water-based makeup.

Oily Skin—Sensitive
This skin type presents some special problems, since proper cleansing requires removal of excess oil but sensitivity precludes the use of strong, vigorously applied cleansers and follow-up products. The following routine has been helpful to many patients with sensitive oily skin.

Morning Cleansing: Wash with a de-greasing but nongranular cleanser such as those suggested for mature oily skin.

Wet your face thoroughly with very warm water, lather up and apply the cleanser with your fingertips. One application is enough. (Do not use physical exfoliators.)

Rinse thoroughly, starting with very warm water, gradually adjusting the temperature to cold.

Follow up with an astringent, toner, or clarifying lotion labeled for oily skin. If these produce a stinging or burning sensation rather than a pleasant tingle, switch to a milder follow-up product, perhaps one labeled for normal skin. Avoid follow-up products containing moisturizing ingredients.

Evening Cleansing: Same as for morning cleansing, but start off with a cream or lotion formulated to dissolve skin oils as it removes water-based makeup.

A few general tips for cleansing oily skin: Do not overdo cleansing. The routines described in this section are designed to be performed twice a day only. To go through any of these routines three, four, or more times a day could leave you with extremely tender, irritated skin. If you feel you need additional de-greasing and cleansing, your skin might be able to tolerate a third washing with mild soap and water; use fingertip application and omit a follow-up product.

Better than washing a third time is to wipe your face occasionally during the day with a special pad saturated with salicylic acid (a good de-greaser) and astringents, such as Therapads Plus.

Do not let magazine or television advertisements talk you into using only cleansing or cold cream to clean your skin. It is true that there are some cream-type products on the market that do a good job of dissolving sebum and removing makeup, and you can use one of them as a first step in evening cleansing. But to look its best your oily skin needs additional soap or detergent de-greasing plus a follow-up product. If you depend solely on a traditional cream-type cleanser, your oily skin will soon be a forest of blackheads and pimples.

Most oily skin benefits from a twice a week treatment with a de-greasing mask containing clay, activated silica, or both. Facial saunas are also good for oily skin. For more on these special treatments, see page 182.

CHAPTER 10

MAKEUP AND OTHER COSMETICS

Cosmetics have changed their image. The ageless art of painting faces and accenting eyes has become the new science of the 1980s. Today's makeup experts are not elegant grande dames; they are lab-coated chemists and technicians, developing and refining the special formulas that promise to color and conceal, refresh and rejuvenate your skin.

Because of the new technology, health has become a watchword in cosmetics these days. For better or worse, many products are now designed to do more than simply cover up; they may contain ingredients to help control mild acne, emollients to avoid dryness, or sunscreens to ward off premature aging and skin cancer. They may be formulated to cooperate with skin medications you are already using. Product lines stress treatment and nourishment over superficial care, while more labels bear high-minded terms such as "moisture balance," "cell renewal," and "oxygen replacement." If many of the claims are highly questionable, more stringent testing and research have at least led to creams and liquids that are less irritating to sensitive skins than ever before.

This new trend toward safe, scientific care may bode well for the consumer, but that is no reason to be complacent. The wrong choice of cosmetic products can aggravate oily, dry, or sensitive skin and possibly trigger a sizable rash or two. Also, certain troublemaking ingredients are still in widespread use. And no matter how thoroughly tested, no product can ever be guaranteed entirely problem-free for everyone.

Basically cosmetics fall into two categories: decorative and (mildly) therapeutic. Those in the first category—most eye and face makeups—will adorn, highlight, or camouflage. What they will not do is physiologically alter your skin or improve an existing condition. Those in the second category may have a below-the-surface effect that relieves certain problems temporarily or changes the skin in some measurable way. Moisturizers, cleansing and wrinkle creams, and even a few face and lip coverups may belong to the latter group.

Regardless of your aim, the best rule of thumb is to choose a cosmetic with the simplest and fewest ingredients. The more complicated the formula, the greater your chances of having a sensitivity reaction (or of paying an unjustifiably inflated price). For example, a so-called medicated or clean cosmetic with dozens of special additives is not necessarily a superior product and it may have a higher potential for irritation and allergic outbreaks. While antiseptic ingredients are useful in lotions that treat minor bruises and cuts, in cosmetics they serve mainly to preserve the product longer rather than to benefit your skin directly in any way.

Cosmetics: The Negative Side

While most cosmetics do their job safely and well, let's turn our attention first to what can go wrong—and why.

A recent joint study of nine thousand families by the Food and Drug Administration and the American Academy of Dermatology found that about eleven percent of cosmetic skin reactions linger long enough to interfere with routine activities. About three percent are sufficiently severe to interrupt them altogether and require a doctor's care. Among the leading sources of trouble are deodorant/antiperspirant products, followed by depilatories, moisturizers, hair sprays, mascaras, bubble bath crystals, eye creams, hair dyes, facial skin creams, lotion cleansers, and nail polishes. While the victims are mostly women, more men are being counted these days, too, as they become avid cosmetic users, especially of lubricants, bronzers, colognes, and aftershave astringents.

Usually sensitivity to cosmetics can be classified as some form of contact dermatitis, a local inflammation that is confined to the site of swelling (non-spreading). Among the symptoms are swelling, redness, burning, bumps, and blisters. A special variety called seborrheic dermatitis can result when cosmetic products combine with the bacteria and oils nesting in the skin to induce an acnelike condition, most often on chin, cheeks and forehead (see Chapter 4).

Certain ingredients may cause reactions only after skin is exposed to the sun, sometimes increasing the chances of severe sunburn. For example, colognes, astringents, and aftershave lotions containing oil of bergamot or extracts of lemon, orange, or lime can all heighten sensitivity to sunlight. Women who dab on perfumes around ears or neck before sunbathing may break out in rashes or burns, which can leave behind a swath of lingering, discolored patches long after the blisters have healed.

When an allergy is involved, skin does not necessarily erupt at the point of contact. Thus, some sensitive nail-polish wearers may end up with swollen, itchy eyelids. (Happily, since nail-polish formulas have been improved in recent years, this reaction is less common today.) An allergy can also arise after long, trouble-free use. Your body's tolerance may change, as you gradually become sensitized over an extended period. Because cosmetics companies are continually changing their formulas slightly, you may even be protesting a new ingredient in your otherwise tried and true product. Perhaps switching to a cosmetic with a higher concentration of a certain raw material will set the stage for trouble.

Not only the user but also a companion can have an allergic reaction: a husband to his wife's hair spray, a child to his father's shaving lotion. To complicate matters further, cosmetics are not the only source of irritated skin. The nickel content in certain costume jewelry, metal eyeglass frames, hairpins, and even brassiere fasteners may spur identical-looking outbreaks and rashes. Occasionally, too, the culprit may be the sponges or brushes used to apply a product, rather than the makeup itself.

Patch testing is one easy, reliable way to determine whether or not you are sensitive to a cosmetic. Apply a small amount to your inner forearm and cover it with an airtight bandage. After one or two days examine the area for any change. Of course, if your skin is already broken, blistered, or irritated, avoid cosmetics entirely: they are intended for use only on clean, healthy skin.

Cosmetics companies are now legally required to list all their products' ingredients in order of weight. But even if you are an avid label reader, the often polysyllabic names may be completely meaningless to you. Those who do manage to crack the cosmetic code will not necessarily learn the quality of the individual parts. You know that a product contains lanolin, for example, but you do not know whether it is high-grade lanolin or lanolin derived from wool wax. And price is no gauge, either. Fancier packaging, advertising, and additives, not superior contents, often account for a product's higher cost.

Fragrances are responsible for more irritation and allergic skin reactions than any other kind of ingredient. Preservatives and dyes follow closely behind as potential troublemakers. Often hundreds of separate elements go into the making of a single fragrance, and none of these are declared on a cosmetic label. However, some dermatologists have samples of known sensitizers for in-office testing, and manufacturers will supply a complete ingredient list for a suspected fragrance at a physician's request to help track down the offender.

Preservatives to avoid include quaternium 15 (responsible for more contact dermatitis than any other ingredient) and formaldehyde. Among common emollients, dimethicone can actually make the skin more absorbent to irritating chemicals, and readily-penetrating isopropyl myristate, often used in foundation creams and lotions, is frequently linked to outbreaks of acne cosmetica (see Chapter 4). Propylene glycol, a widely used humectant (water-attracting agent) in moisturizing creams, can cause allergic reactions in sensitive skins.

Some cosmetic materials are not benign but rather biologically active chemicals that may enter the bloodstream with possibly harmful effects if used over a long period of time. For example, while the estrogens in anti-wrinkle creams have been reduced as a result of studies linking hormones with cancer of the uterine lining, even small amounts can be absorbed and have a cumulative effect. Chemical preservatives are sometimes contaminated with substances called nitrosamines (potentially cancer-causing agents), including TEA and DEA and the preservative 2-bromo-2-nitropropane-1, 3-diol (BNPD).

D&C red #9 and D&C red #19, two dyes used in lipsticks, have also been cited as possible cancer inducers. And two other dyes, D&C red #21 and #27, especially abundant in the so-called indelible lipsticks, can cause cheiltis in about ten percent of users, a condition marked by drying, cracking, blistering, swelling, and burning. Other reactions to concentrated lip dyes include excessive tearing, hives, dermatitis, and even severe nasal congestion. Symptoms disappear about two weeks after the product is discontinued. ("D&C" means that the color has been approved for use in drugs and cosmetics but not for use in food. "Ext. D&C" means approved for external application only, not for use on lips or mucous membranes.)

While some cosmetic dyes, such as chlorophyll and carotene, are of natural origin, most are derived from substances called soluble coal tars. These have been the subject of controversy, because they are a fairly common source of allergy and have led to tumors when injected into the skins of mice. As of now, six are considered safe; others are presently on the Food and Drug Administration's provisional list, which means that proof of their safety has yet to be confirmed. (Some have had this dubious status for more than twenty years!)

Face powders and blushers are among the least troublesome cosmetics, although some may attract bacterial growth if kept too long or used incorrectly. As for liquid foundations, these are basically mixtures of water, oils, and pigment in varying concentrations. Although many oil bases create a fertile breeding ground for acne, these may sometimes (paradoxically) be less irritating than stronger, water-soluble, completely oil-free ingredients such as the detergents used in foundations formulated for oily or normal skin. Trial and error rather than a label claim is the best way to judge whether a product is appropriate for your skin.

Cosmetic Creams and Lotions

Let's examine the cosmetics that have more than a simple decorative function.

Most facial cleansing creams are simply a combination of oils, waxes, and water, and based on the standard cold cream formula first published nearly two thousand years ago by a Greek physician. (The natural oil base dissolves other greasy substances, namely heavy makeup.) Despite manufacturers' boasts about their products containing no harsh soaps, the more sophisticated varieties often include strong de-greasers and detergents such as sodium lauryl sulfate, along with assorted emollients (skin softeners) and humectants (water-attracting ingredients). These extras raise both the cost and the risk of irritation without adding any substantial benefit.

Astringents, also known as fresheners, toners, and pore lotions, are cleansing products that help dissolve oils and remove makeup. Common alcohol, the main ingredient, temporarily tightens the pores and causes a tingling sensation. It is often mixed with a natural plant extract, such as witch hazel. Any other additives, such as the lubricants, colorings, and fragrances contained in the more elaborate formulas, contribute little except to the price (and possibly sex appeal).

The same rule of simplicity applies to moisturizers. Skin becomes dry as a result of losing moisture, not oil, so it is moisture that must be replenished. Thus, the purpose of a moisturizer is simply to lock in water and natural fluids with a thin coating of oil or grease. The end result is to plump up the skin's thirsty outer cells and smooth out the rough, scaly surface. Almost any oil or grease will do, and it makes sense to apply moisturizer only after shower or bath, when the skin is slightly damp.

Despite the dizzying array of claims, most of the ingredients in high-priced formulas have little to do with moisturizing. A few may actually irritate sensitive skin, an effect that may not be obvious immediately, since all creams and lotions temporarily mask dry skin problems. So far, only two substances have been proven scientifically to be of lasting benefit: lanolin and petrolatum, two basic, inexpensive raw materials. When applied twice daily for three weeks, these were shown to ward off dryness in test subjects for up to three weeks after being discontinued. Of course, in their unvarnished state, both ingredients lack the elegance and aesthetic appeal of other formulas. (Their greasiness can be minimized by a dusting of talc or baby powder.) In addition, a small percentage of people are allergic to raw lanolin, and the higher grades (such as the acetylated kind) may be too pore-clogging for those with acne or oily skin. Thick, greasy petrolatum, too, can be equally acnegenic.

The next most beneficial products are water-in-oil emulsions. Those with more oil than water are creams, while those with more water than oil are lotions. Creams are more potent barriers against moisture loss. Eucerin and Nivea creams are prime examples of effective agents. The best-acting moisturizers also have hydrophilic properties—they combine with water rather than separate from it. Smear some of the preparation in the palm of your hand, add a few drops of water, and rub. If the liquid readily disappears, the product is hydrophilic. Good no-frills remedies include Hydrophilic Ointment USP (a salve, four parts ointment, one part water), urea (available as a 10 percent or 20 percent product under various brand names), and mineral oil. These are ideal for all skin types—light, inexpensive, and essentially non-occlusive.

Formulas with a high glycerin content also work well, particularly in humid climates, since this ingredient attracts moisture from the air to hydrate the skin. (In dry environments, pure glycerin has the opposite effect, drawing water away from the outer layers. But most glycerin products are at least fifty percent water, so they will not dry out your skin, even in Arizona.)

Since any oil and water base is a perfect haven for bacteria, preservatives are necessary ingredients in all commercial moisturizers. The more sophisticated mixtures also contain emulsifiers to keep creams and lotions soft and of the right consistency—to make the product "spreadable" longer. Just as with other cosmetics, however, perfumes, colorings, and thickeners are superfluous and costly additives in any moisturizer or cleansing cream.

Guidelines: How to Be Safe
and Savvy

Aside from lists of ingredients, cosmetic labels often include certain giveaway words. "Sheer," "natural," "translucent," "matte," and "velvety" generally denote nongreasy or water-based products best suited to oily skin, while "moist," "dewy," "good coverup," and "enriched formula" signal an oil-based product. Almost every product today carries a claim that it is greaseless, but even the blatant term "oil-free" is often misleading; cosmetics so labeled may be irritating enough to trigger acne. To tell whether oil is present, use the blotting paper test described in Chapter 4.

The reassuring terms "dermatologist-tested," "hypoallergenic," and "clinically formulated" technically mean a product is less likely to cause a sensitivity reaction—a claim that generally carries a higher selling price. Usually products labeled this way are made without fragrances and certain oils, so to minimize their potential for irritation. But so have many other cosmetics, which do not bear such fancy seals of approval—or the heftier price tags to match. So do not be too readily swayed by scientific-sounding terms. Decide whether the added cost is really worth it.

To keep problems to a minimum, observe any reactions in your skin after using cosmetics and do not hesitate to discard a product at the first sign of irritation. If a product comes with directions on package or insert, follow these carefully.

Get well acquainted with your skin and choose cosmetics that are most compatible with your type. Reevaluate your skin's profile every six months or so, since changes in environment or levels of stress may alter your needs. Use the guidelines in Chapter 1 to help you identify key strengths and weaknesses. Alternatively, rely on trained department-store personnel for an evaluation. Have your skin tested at more than one counter and ask how the conclusions were arrived at. (This service is free of charge, entailing no obligation to buy a given company's products.)

When considering a purchase, don't ever be oversold. Chances are that you need only one or two products rather than a whole treatment line. Ask questions to help you pinpoint the most appropriate cosmetic—for example, whether the alcohol content in a moisturizer is high enough for your oily skin, whether a foundation is oil-, water-, or alcohol-based. If you have very sensitive skin, test dime-sized samples on your inner forearm (then wait a day or two) before buying, and avoid mixing products from different companies, since ingredients may clash, possibly with irritating effects. (The components of one product line have at least been designed to work together compatibly.)

Wash your hands well before using cosmetics and keep lids and containers tightly sealed. Every time you open a jar or use your fingers on a product, you introduce a host of microorganisms, all potentially infection-carriers. For maximum freshness, buy cream-based cosmetics in small quantities—only as much as you will use in six months. To retard spoilage during the summer, keep them refrigerated rather than exposed to the bathroom's heat and humidity.

Be extra cautious when applying cosmetics around the eyes. Most problems related to eye makeup, particularly mascara—a rigorously tested category—stem from using applicators carelessly, sharing, swapping, or failing to clean brushes (perfect hiding places for bacteria), moistening dried or cake products with saliva (a practice that can result in serious infection), keeping products too long before discarding them, or applying the makeup in a moving vehicle. Choose only products labeled for use in the area of the eyes and be sure they are clean and well covered. If irritation develops, see a doctor immediately.

Remember Shakespeare's advice: Neither a borrower nor a lender be. An epidemic of trachoma, a disease that can blind, erupted at a girls' school after eyeliners were shared.

If you have any complaints or inquiries regarding cosmetics—if you believe the labeling is wrong or misleading, if directions for use are unclear, or if you have an adverse reaction—report it both to the manufacturers and to the Food and Drug Administration. Write to:

Food and Drug Administration
Division of Cosmetics Technology, HFF-430
200 C Street, S.W.
Washington, D.C. 20204

In 1979, the Food and Drug Administration asked cosmetic houses to submit voluntary reports confirming the safety of their products. And right now a panel of independent scientists is attempting to review key ingredients and evaluate them for risk. Observers hope that this will pave the way for official government guidelines (at last!) about what should and should not be in cosmetic products.

Cosmetics: The Ultimate Con Game?

Behind every high-priced cosmetic lurks an image. The most prestigious companies spend untold sums trying to persuade us that their products are unique, exotic, ultraglamorous. And high price is part of the package, a carefully calculated ploy designed to convince us that we are buying something very special. After all, a costly item carries class and one that "promises fantasy must be priced fantastically" as well, a witty observer notes. Even the most seasoned consumers associate greater expense with superior quality.

So, according to the rules of image, elegant salons and chic department stores are the most favored outlets for these luxury wares. Selling at discount is discouraged, and cut-rate merchants are deliberately snubbed. In fact, some companies will not sell their cosmetics directly to any discount store.

Do you really get what you pay for? A recent five-part series on the CBS Evening News raised the question and uncovered some surprising answers.

When asked what makes their product line so special and why their cosmetics are unfailingly expensive, a spokesman for a high-prestige firm pointed to the range and quality of their colors. "We offer the richest, most dazzling palette," he claimed, and proudly cited a luscious shade of blusher as the company's hottest-selling item. But researchers discovered that a discount house sells the very same blusher under a different name for exactly half the price. Both color and ingredients are identical. Because the company spends less on advertising and uses a cheaper package, it can afford to sell its cosmetics for less.

The discount firm declined to reveal more inside information, so CBS newsmen were forced to go undercover for a more thorough explanation. Posing as buyers, a makeup artist and a producer (equipped with a hidden tape recorder) set out for a major cosmetics factory in Long Island City. There a salesman led them into a showroom filled with samples of the factory's stock colors. The CBS investigators were told they could buy any of the colors for 18 cents and put their own label on a package. Would they then have the very same product as the high-priced brands? they asked. Yes, was the immediate response; the factory did not vary any of the ingredients, regardless of the client. What spelled the difference was simply packaging, promotion, and, of course, the selling price. A half-ounce of eye shadow bought directly from the factory costs about $1. The major companies, of course, do not want their secret to be common knowledge. One calls its products "exclusive"; others insist their formulas are "special."

But the Long Island firm reports that all these companies and others buy their cosmetics there, each one whipped up from the same standard colors and formulas. Thus, the trade name for one expensive house's best-selling color is Big Apple Blush—advertised in the factory catalogue at a wholesale price of 40¢! The same holds true for mascara. A 60¢ item is sold by one non-advertised company for $3.50 and in a smaller bottle by the well-known firm for $5.50.

Since the products are identical, what counts above all is image—discount blisterpacks versus elegant showcases at expensive department stores. Which product seems more seductive, more exotic? Which suggests higher status? The answer is all in an artful sales pitch, an aura of sophistication and luxury conveyed by the right words and wrappings.

From another factory in Fairlawn, New Jersey, the television investigators heard a very similar story—cheap and expensive often emerge from the very same vat. Also, topline companies will often cut back on distribution, making their product harder to get, so that it will simply seem more valuable. While deliberately selling less sounds like a curious way to do business, ultimately it is profitable, since scarcity suggests exclusivity, and most people are willing to pay the price.

For their New Jersey venture, the CBS team posed as businessmen seeking to start their own cosmetics line. They discovered that an equally prestigious roster of companies is serviced by this factory, which manufactures lipstick, mascara, creams, liquid makeup, face powder, and eyeshadow from raw material to finished product—everything except nail polish and deodorant, as the factory president explains. A case in point is a discount brand of lipstick (called Wilson), which retails for about $3; it contains exactly the same colors and ingredients as its more than twice as expensive counterpart. The New Jersey manufacturers say the formula is theirs.

Incidentally, the factory sells Wilson's plastic case for 40¢ and the metal "famous" case for 45¢. The lipstick itself costs about 35¢, less than the container it comes in. When one company wants another's color, the company just orders it from the factory and then markets it under a different name. Sometimes the very same vat of lipstick is divided into different companies' shipments.

The newsmen found that the biggest profits can be made on creams and moisturizers. It is easy to sell a $1 jar for $25, presumably because the promise of instant youthfulness is the most enticing one of all. (But for smoothing and softening dry or wrinkled skin, plain mineral oil is just as effective as the fanciest hormone cream.) To make their formula "unique," companies sometimes pressure cosmetic chemists to add an exotic but unnecessary ingredient or group of additives, which neither enhances nor detracts from the original recipe. What this does is to give the company a story angle for their copywriters and yet another rationale for a puffed-up price.

One final note: The CBS on-air reporter revealed that he and his staff had been researching this exposé for twelve straight weeks and yet had managed to find only one cosmetic chemist who was willing to talk to them. They even visited universities without success. When asked for information, one professor bluntly replied that his department was generously funded by industry and he could not risk offending it. So the continuing silence keeps most consumers in the dark, misled by fanciful claims and clever promotional devices. The CBS crew learned the facts only because they went underground and because one (retired) cosmetic chemist was willing to speak out.

Patricia Boughton and Marcia Ellen Hughes, authors of *The Buyer's Guide to Cosmetics,* agree that price matters little when the quality of cosmetics is being judged, but found two exceptions. Their own survey revealed that the more expensive brands of liquid foundations and mascaras were generally rated higher by consumers for their consistency, durability, and naturalness. On the whole, they conclude that differences in price often boil down to degrees of aesthetic appeal, varying textures, and different methods of application. Their suggestion is to sample a wide variety of price ranges and formulas first. Only then can you decide whether eye-catching extras and name-brand prestige are worth the added expense.

The Art: How to Apply Makeup

In Renaissance Europe, the portrait painters of the court were also makeup artists. They adorned the features of their noble subjects with cosmetics just as they flattered them with the skillful use of the palette. Like a pleasing portrait, the right makeup casts your face in the very best light and makes it look chiseled, well contoured, free of flaws and rough spots. "The purpose of makeup is to play certain areas up or down, to alter or accent bone structure, and to smooth out texture and tone," explains Bert Roth, director of makeup at ABC-TV. The proper colors can add rosy warmth to sallow skin or soften an overly ruddy complexion. Narrow faces can be widened and round ones made longer and more angular, so that both appear perfect ovals.

The basic tools for refining and changing the appearance of skin are foundations, powders, blushers, eye makeups, and lip colors. Dark-shaded pencils and powders tend to make areas of the face recede or look smaller, while light tones emphasize or enlarge them. Ideally, cosmetics should form a perfect illusion; they should be applied so artfully and subtly that not even the most attentive observer can tell where they begin or end.

Start by making sure skin is thoroughly cleaned and hair is tied back. While face is still damp, apply a moisturizer if your skin type requires it. Then cover dark circles and unevenly pigmented areas or blemishes with an opaque masking cream or coverstick one shade lighter than your skin tone. Next dab on liquid, cream, or powder foundation, smoothing a bit first onto your jawline in a bright light and blending well to make sure the color matches your skin. Too dark a shade will seem muddy, while too light will give you a masklike, painted look. With your fingertips dot liquid or cream on the middle of your forehead, under your eyes, on nose, cheeks, and chin. Blend it evenly in a clockwise direction. Apply a circle of blusher cream or powder (smiling broadly to help you place it correctly), then smooth on in an upward movement from cheek to temple.

Too much blusher or too dark a shade tends to give cheekbones a flattened look. For most natural results, add a hint of color along cheekbones, at the edge of your forehead, on the bridge of your nose, even on earlobes. For more definition, you might add a contouring (darker) shade at the bottom edge of your cheekbones. To help set color longer, pat on a powder rouge first, then cover with a cream rouge of the same shade (or vice versa). Oily-skinned women who prefer a drier look should fluff on a colorless translucent powder before brushing on rouge. (Applying the latter directly over moist foundation will lead to caking.)

To add some bone structure to a rounded face, after adding blush, make a light crescent on your cheekbones (about a fingertip below the outer corner of each eye) with a foundation or coverstick one or two shades lighter than your skin, then blend well. To add width to a narrow face, blend blusher in a straight line from the outer half of each cheek to middle of ear.

To make a double chin disappear, cover it with a foundation or powder three to four shades darker than your skin tone (remember, darkness de-emphasizes) and blend well toward ears. Conversely, build up a receding chin by covering it with a lighter makeup.

If your nose is too long, place shadow (a shade or two darker than your foundation) under the tip to make it appear shorter. Blend carefully to avoid a soiled look and dust over with powder to seal the results. To narrow or play down a too-broad shape, apply light makeup down the center of your nose and shadow the sides, blending very carefully and finishing off with powder.

According to most makeup artists, your eyebrows should extend from the inner to the outer corner of the eye, with the highest point of the arch directly above the outermost part of the iris. Regard them as a frame rather than a focal point. Overtweezed eyebrows look unexpressive, while overly bushy or emphatic eyebrows draw too much attention away from the eyes. If eyes are close-set, widen the space between the eyebrows a bit by trimming the ends above the inner corner of the eyes and extending the other ends slightly with a pencil. If eyes are too far apart, bring eyebrows closer to the nose with a coloring pencil.

Light eyeshadows on the lids will make deep-set eyes come forward; darker tones will minimize a bulging or pop-eyed look. For eyes too far apart, darker shadows at the inner corner of the lids and lighter colors at the outer end will bring them closer together. (Just the opposite holds for close-set eyes, of course.) For lids that are too heavy, lighter shades work best, blended with a slightly darker shadow on the crease above. To prevent smudging (caused by friction due to blinking, not oils, since glands are virtually absent here), make powder eyeshadows your first choice and never use an eye cream or moisturizer beneath.

Eyeshadow has changed with the times. Today it is

considered too obvious and contrived to smear the lid with one horizontal block of color; the contemporary look calls for the use of more than one shade. For example, a striking green may be brushed on the outer corner to draw the eye outward, with a soft brown on the inner corner to add depth. The colors should be subtly blended, one into the other. Shadow should be paler between the lashes and the fold of the lid than in the space between the crease and eyebrow. For evening, a more dramatic yet still natural look is in. Try a coppery shadow on the lid, softened with a bit of brown in the corner of the eye and above the crease. Smudge some ginger or another warm spice color just above the lashes for added interest. Just remember, no matter how many different shades you use, none should be distinctly definable.

To add verve and width to eyes at any time of day, draw a line with white pencil or light-blue eyeliner along the rim just inside the lower eyelashes.

As for lips, to prevent color from bleeding or wandering, outline your mouth first with a non-greasy pencil a shade or two darker than your lipstick (making thin lips wider or full lips narrower, if you choose). Then, using a brush, fill in the outline with your chosen lip color. Blot with a tissue and reapply. For a more muted look, finish off with a white.

To help makeup stay on longer, dust foundation with loose translucent powder (a fluffy brush is best), then dip a fine sponge in ice-cold water, squeeze well, and pat over face.

General color guide: Greens and blues offset ruddiness, pink and pale rose enliven a whitish, sallow look, and mauve tones correct an olive complexion. Keep in mind that green or bluish fluorescent lighting may wash out color somewhat and accentuate acne and shadows, calling for a slightly bolder touch. On the other hand, more muted shades will suffice under natural outdoor or daylight-simulating fluorescent light.

The Changing Face of Makeup

No cosmetic routine is ever fixed for all time. What flatters at one age may seem too subtle or bold a few years later. This is because skin is a constantly changing organ, as weather, sun, and time leave their traces at every decade.

The general rule is: Wear the least makeup in your teens when skin is at its oiliest, use more in your twenties and thirties to moisturize and conceal, and sport a more conservative look again in your forties, fifties, and beyond. As you enter your thirties, for example, you might choose to switch from a powder to a cream or vice versa, or find that the frosted, slick-surfaced looks you have always prized suddenly throw a spotlight on fine lines and imperfections.

Here are some guidelines.

Teens
If skin is afflicted with acne, conceal blemishes first with skin-toned drying preparations containing sulfur or resorcinol or both, blending well. Then apply a very light film of oil-free or water-based foundation with a damp sponge. Dust lightly all over with a non-comedogenic translucent powder (made without the troublesome ingredients listed under "Acne Cosmetica" in Chapter 4) and follow with a naturally drying gel or powder blush rather than a cream-based product. Use moisturizers only if skin is especially dry, such as after washing or spending a day in the sun or blustery cold. If skin is invariably dry, taut,

and free of acne, you can choose any foundation that looks best and moisturize more liberally.

Note: Avoid plucking eyebrows too zealously, since you may damage delicate follicles and pave the way for sparser growth later on.

Twenties

While acne generally tones down during this decade, heavier use of cosmetics along with plain workaday stress may set off a new explosion.

A non-greasy foundation followed by translucent powder is still the ideal choice, though dust it very lightly over any dry patches of skin. If skin is still oily, use powder or gel blushers to prevent colors from fading too easily. Otherwise, you may use cream blushers instead (though always beware of irritating, acne-prodding ingredients. Consult the list in Chapter 4.). Be conservative with moisturizers, applying only when your skin or surroundings are especially dry. (Wet the skin first for best results, of course.) However, when using color, do not hesitate to be dramatic and experimental, if your prefer, particularly with eye and lip products; choose shades from any side of the spectrum.

Thirties

While a liberal use of colors and textures applies for this age group also, the possible debut of fine lines, larger pores, or both may call for a slight shift in strategy. Strive for a mat look in eyeshadows and foundations, since shine and glitter only highlight fine lines and creases. Use gentle moisturizers after cleansing and also to help set makeup more effectively.

Forties

The key to natural looks at this age is a light touch.

Powders or creams applied too liberally will only collect in creases and folds, accenting rather than concealing them. The mat, dry-faced look is desirable, since shine magnifies flaws. This holds true for lipsticks and eye makeups, too; high-gloss, pearly types can point up even the finest lines.

When blending upward and outward, avoid brushing powder blusher into crow's-feet and do not extend it too far below the cheekbone, either, where it may overlap with a smile line or two. Cake eyeliners (moistened with water) reflect light more evenly and are less likely to collect in wrinkles and crepey folds at this stage.

Heavy night-creams around the eyes may retain moisture so effectively that they lead to morning puffiness.

Eyebrows may need more emphasis at this age, since hair growth begins to slow down.

Fifties and Beyond

The hormonal shifts caused by menopause result in drier, less elastic facial skin and sometimes a crop of coarser hairs around chin and upper lip. At this time, age or liver spots may also appear on the face and anywhere else that has been much exposed to the sun.

While cream-based foundations are probably the best concealers, be sure to apply them sparingly, since creams (along with gels) tend to sink into folds and creases rather than remain on the surface as powders do. Whatever foundation you choose, stick with powder blushers and eyeshadows for the most natural results.

Avoid bright colors on both eyes and lips—these give faces a painted, clownish look—and select muted shades and softer neutrals instead, especially if hair is gray or graying. In general, downplay any kind of makeup, since excess only exaggerates defects.

Watch out for moles that change in size, shape, or color, along with sunspots (keratoses) and the scaly patches of seborrheic dermatitis. These are problems that call for a dermatologists's care.

Facial Masks

When used occasionally, these highly touted cosmetic
items can be soothing yet stimulating supplements to regular
cleansing. But you do not need masks any more than you
need bubble baths or strawberry-flavored lipsticks. They
simply feel good and lift your spirits; do not expect them
to "deep cleanse" your pores (the term is meaningless),
clear away acne, or do anything beyond toning the skin
temporarily.

Masks usually harden on contact with the skin and are
designed to be left on the face and neck (avoid the delicate
eye area) from ten to twenty minutes. During this interval
the mask will improve circulation and cleanse the skin of
surface greasiness. Masks are removed by being peeled off
or rinsed with lukewarm water. Skin will appear fresher,
cleaner, softer, because masks lift away dead, scaly cells,
dirt, and makeup. Also gently stimulating for both hands
and feet, masks have a pleasant aftereffect and improve
overall skin texture.

Some makeup artists believe that masks prime the surface of the skin, making it more receptive to cosmetics and
more radiant in color. The rosy flush may fade after
several hours, while the smooth, silken feeling may linger
for one or two days. For oilier skin, clay-based formulas
are generally recommended, while moisturizing vegetable
or herbal varieties are considered more suitable for drier
skin. Unless you follow up with an oil or cream, however,
the moisture will evaporate, leaving your skin drier than
before. (Beauty experts believe that steaming your face

beforehand will enable you to derive the maximum benefit from any mask.)

There is no need to take yourself to an exclusive health spa or facial salon to enjoy this luxury. The following are some suggestions from Aida Grey, Inc., on the very best homemade formulas for different types of skin.

Dry Skin

- Mash 1 medium-sized banana (preferably not too ripe), add 1 tablespoon honey, mix well. Leave on for 15 minutes. Remove with tepid water.
- Blend 1 egg yolk and 1 tablespoon honey until smooth. Leave on for 15 minutes. Remove with tepid water.
- For dry and sallow skin, ½ cup sour cream. Leave on for 30 minutes. Remove with tepid water.

Normal or Combination Skin

- Dissolve 3 tablespoons honey in 2 tablespoons boiling water. Add 2 teaspoons lemon juice and mix well until a paste is formed. Leave on for 20 minutes. Remove with tepid water.
- Beat 2 egg yolks until frothy and light-colored, add 1 teaspoon apricot oil, blend until smooth. Add 1 teaspoon lemon juice and mix well. Leave on for 20 minutes. Remove with tepid water.
- Combine 1/3 cup ground almonds with enough witch hazel to form a paste. Leave on for 15 minutes. Remove with tepid water.
- Combine 1 sliced, medium-sized peeled apple, 1 tablespoon honey, and 1 tablespoon skim milk in a blender. Leave on for 20 minutes.

Oily Skin

- Combine 2 beaten egg whites, 1 tablespoon nonfat dry milk, and 1 teaspoon honey. Blend to form a paste.

Leave on for 20 minutes. Remove with tepid water.

• Grate a small unpeeled potato. Place the gratings in gauze and apply to the face, then cover with absorbent cotton dipped in milk. Leave on for 20 minutes. Rinse with tepid water.

• Mix 1 cake brewer's yeast (or 1 packet active dry yeast) with enough mineral water to form a paste. Leave on for 30 minutes. Remove with warm water.

What Rates Best

A recent test conducted by *Family Circle* concludes that excellent cosmetics, many priced at under $3, are available in supermarkets and discount stores. More than five hundred women sampled products from seventy-five of the leading cosmetics companies. The following budget-priced items were their top choices.

L'Erin Moisture Fresh Liquid Makeup: Liquid foundation in eight shades. Testers reported that it provides transparent, natural-looking coverage and a smooth, mat finish, wears well, and is easy to remove.

Johnson's Baby Powder: Loose white powder in a plastic container with shaker top. Testers said it makes a superb face powder when fluffed lightly over makeup.

Cover Girl Brush-On Blush: Powder blush. Comes with a brush applicator but no mirror, in bright colors, pink to bronze. Testers said it buffs up to a warm, flattering glow, natural colors, and a dry, mat texture, is non-irritating and easily removable.

Bonne Bell Colorado Colors Eyeshadow Duo: Powder shadow. Comes in a mirror compact with sponge-tip applicator, two contrasting colors, one mat and one iridescent, per compact. Testers said the product is long-lasting, easily applied, and has a smooth finish.

Sally Hansen Perfect Lips: Clear and colored gloss with wand applicator. Testers liked it better than all other glosses, used alone or over lipstick, reporting that it gives a high shine and a popular wet look. The wand applicator is said to be well designed, with an unusually small, slanted tip for easy application.

Maybelline Fresh Lash Mascara: Liquid polymer mascara. Waterproof and comes in three shades. Testers rated it excellent for ease of application, color, durability, and applicator design.

CHAPTER 11

SAVE FACE AND LOSE WEIGHT: THE HEALTHY SKIN DIET

An attractive face and body are much more than skin deep. They start with what you eat. A nutritionally wholesome diet provides the energy that fuels your constantly renewed cells. It nourishes the network of blood vessels, nerves, and fibers that give shape and substance to your skin. And it maintains your miraculous internal cleansing machine by carrying off impurities that can lead to a blemished, lackluster surface.

The key words for any skin-smart eating plan are "moderation" and "consistency." Overfeeding your body may well result in starving your skin. A diet too high in fats and oils, refined sugars, starches, and otherwise empty calories can lead to a buildup of fatty materials beneath the surface. This excess may constrict the tiny capillaries that carry nutrients and moisture to the outer skin. The consequence is a complexion robbed of vitality and healthy tone. Too much salt and adulterated or artificial ingredients can cause fluid retention and bloated, puffy skin.

If you diet, avoid the so-called yo-yo syndrome—losing and regaining pounds in rapid succession. Sudden, dramatic shifts in weight and eating habits or a chronic calorie deficit can upset the body's delicate metabolism, with all too visible impact on your skin. For example, a number of people on the notorious liquid protein diet complained of persistent cracking and flaking, even months after they went off the drastic regimen. Worse, almost any crash program may end up leaving a permanent legacy of sags, stretch marks, and wrinkles. Why? If you shed more than three or four pounds a week, your body mass will shrink faster than the normally elastic skin can reshape itself to accommodate it.

Another diet taboo is skipping meals or eating on the run, which can result in overcompensating later on. Studies have shown that you will lose weight more effectively by eating three square meals a day than by fitting your allotted calories into only one or two meals. Eat slowly, savoring every bite, and try to do it at a regularly designated time and place. Rushing and mindlessly gulping can encourage overeating, since the brain requires at least twenty minutes to relay the signal that the stomach is full and satisfied. Also, nervous tension interferes with the digestion and circulation of nutrients.

The effects of a poor or inadequate diet can show up in a variety of unattractive ways, from pallor, rashes, and scaling to easy bruising and lack of resilience. Certain vitamin and nutrient deficiencies—potentially a problem for chronic dieters—can spur specific skin disorders. Sagging skin and stretch marks may be hastened by a shortage of protein or certain trace elements, especially zinc and copper, or by a lack of vitamin C. Too little riboflavin (B_2) can lead to excessive oiliness and cracking, sores, or a whitening of the skin around the mouth; a low level of B_6 has been linked to scaling and seborrhea; and a niacin deficiency may result in dermatitis.

Some nutritionists believe that over fifty percent of the food you eat should be in its whole, uncooked, natural state. That means raw (or lightly steamed) vegetables, high-fiber grains, and fresh, unpeeled fruits instead of packaged snack foods and sweet desserts.

Skin is largely protein- and calcium-based, and we keep it fresh, smooth, and problem-free by feeding it more of the same. Most Americans are probably overnourished with protein, but much of it is in the form of foods too high in saturated fats. Concentrate on fish, legumes (beans and peas), unrefined whole grains, and low-fat dairy products, along with poultry and the leanest cuts of meat, preferably broiled, baked, braised, or stir-fried, oriental style. Inadequate protein for long periods of time (a possible result of unsupervised fasting or fad dieting) can contribute to a loss of elasticity and tone, a slower rate of healing, and premature wrinkling. Many protein-rich foods also contain iron, which the skin needs for healthy color and adequate moisture. Iron deficiency anemia can show up as extreme paleness, dryness, and even hair loss. As for calcium, the best sources include dairy foods (preferably the low-fat kind), sardines, broccoli, green leafy vegetables, kidney beans, and a mineral supplement which provides calcium and magnesium in a roughly two to one ratio.

Feeding Your Skin

Here, in brief, is what the major nutrients can do for your skin. Think of them as pieces of a puzzle which all have to interlock to make a finished picture. Of course, no single element is a miracle ingredient that can restore or guarantee good health or ensure a vibrant, glowing complexion. But just as no jigsaw is complete until every piece is in place, even one nutritional missing link can leave a telltale mark on your skin.

Vitamin A
Recent studies suggest that vitamin A preserves elasticity

and smoothness, staves off dryness, and helps delay the aging and wrinkling process. A chronic A deficiency may result in thickening of the outer layers, blocked oil glands, flakiness, itching, or a goose-bump texture on the surface of the skin. It may also pose a higher risk of epithelial cancer, which can appear in the skin, lungs, cervix, and gastrointestinal tract.

Golden-fleshed fruits and yellow vegetables, such as apricots, peaches, squash, carrots, and yams, are among the best natural sources of A, along with calves' liver and the much-maligned fish liver oils. Dark, leafy greens— parsley, spinach, romaine, and watercress—are good providers, too. (If you are taking dietary supplements of vitamin A, be aware that excessive amounts over a long period of time can have possible toxic effects.)

The B Complex

This indispensable group is essential for smooth, glossy, blemish-free skin. Whole-grain breads and cereals, legumes, green vegetables, brewer's yeast (a virtual storehouse of Bs), eggs, yogurt, lean meats, bananas, and brown rice are excellent sources.

Since the B-complex vitamins are water-soluble, they are not stored by the body and have to be replenished daily. They are also easily lost to heat during cooking. So taking a balanced supplement can help ensure an adequate amount.

Being on the Pill can increase your requirement for B_6 and folic acid (another B factor) by as much as ten times. Alcohol and drugs are also notorious B robbers.

Vitamin C

This extremely important nutrient cooperates with protein to form the collagen "glue" and elastin tissue essential for youthful, well-toned skin. Evidence indicates that vitamin C enhances the body's ability to absorb and use iron and may also counteract the effects of nitrosamines, potential cancer-causing agents in the body. Furthermore, C is crucial to strong, elastic blood-vessel walls and healthy cell membranes, both major components of skin.

Citrus fruits, strawberries, tomatoes, potatoes, leafy greens (especially watercress, parsley, and turnip greens), broccoli, cabbage, and kale are good natural sources, but some nutritionists and physicians advise supplementing the diet with at least 500 to 1,000 mgs. a day of this volatile, water-soluble vitamin (preferably in a buffered tablet form).

A whole orange is more nutritious than freshly squeezed juice. The inner skin and membranes of the fruit contain both vitamin C and bioflavonoids, which are essential for sturdy capillaries.

Vitamin D
The well-known "sunshine" vitamin is needed to help transport and utilize the calcium in our system, which is necessary for the functioning of the nerves, blood vessels, and muscles and the maintenance of sturdy teeth and bones. Salmon, sardines, herring, eggs, fortified dairy products, and liver are all primary sources.

Vitamin E
This nutrient is believed to keep you younger-looking by helping to retard the aging of cells brought about by the interaction of oxygen with other chemicals in the body. It also maintains and preserves cell membranes of the major organs. Vegetable oils, wheat germ, brewer's yeast, whole-grain breads and cereals, leafy greens, soybeans, and eggs are among the best sources. Daily supplements of 100 to 200 IUs are being advised by a growing number of physicians.

Vitamin K
Yet another staple, this nutrient facilitates blood-clotting.

Insufficient amounts may lead to increased bruising of the skin and a slower rate of healing. Normally the body produces what it needs from the bacteria present in the small intestine. When you are taking antibiotics, which upset the natural intestinal flora, supplement with extra vitamin K by increasing your intake of green leafy vegetables.

Other key nutrients are:

Zinc
Recently scientists have discovered that this versatile mineral can speed the healing process after a cut or burn, possibly help clear pimples, foster the production and growth of new cells, and aid in the formation of skin proteins. The British medical journal *Lancet* reported that a group of patients with chronic boils showed unusually low levels of zinc, but after a month of daily supplements, their boils vanished without a recurrence.

To ensure a plentiful supply of zinc, eat mostly unadulterated, wholesome foods—beans, seeds, peas, whole grains (especially wheat germ, wheat bran, and brewer's yeast), lamb, pork, chicken, and seafood, particularly oysters, lobster, and crabmeat. A daily supplement of 20 to 30 mgs. is considered safe and acceptable.

Essential Fatty Acids (EFA)
Available in nuts, seeds, cereal grains, corn and safflower oils, these also play a leading role in skin cell growth and renewal.

Sulfur
When proteins are broken down into amino acids, which are then reassembled into substances that are usable by the body, sulfur is a key ingredient or catalyst in this process. You will find plenty in the aromatic foods, such as cab-

bage, cauliflower, brussels sprouts, onion, garlic, and egg yolks.

Iron

This familiar staple is needed for a healthy blood supply (which shows up as a rosy color) and the prevention of anemia, hair loss, and dryness. Get your daily quota from nuts, whole grains, leafy greens, legumes, liver, shellfish, and egg yolks, along with the amount available in a good vitamin/mineral supplement. (Raw spinach is not a good source, because it contains oxalic acid, which binds the iron and prevents its absorption by the body.)

Watch out for:

Overcooking

Remember, whenever possible fruits and vegetables should be eaten raw or else cooked minimally—steamed or stir-fried or boiled for short periods in small amounts of water. Save the cooking water for soups and stews to get the full benefit of all nutrients. And do not store fresh produce or fruit juices for more than a few days in the refrigerator, as these lose vitamins rapidly.

Drinking

The best beverage for your skin is water, straight from the tap (equipped with a filter) or, preferably, a bottled, low-sodium kind such as Poland Springs or plain seltzer. Drink generously to keep skin well lubricated from within. Beware of diet sodas while you are losing weight; they are relatively sodium-rich, which leads to bloating from fluid retention, and in some people they can act as photosensitizers—intensifying sun damage and possibly leaving dark blotches on the skin later on.

Too much alcohol is doubly destructive. It interferes

with the absorption of B vitamins, so crucial for healthy skin, and dilates the blood vessels, particularly on the face. (Other foods, such as chili, caffeine, curried Indian dishes, Szechuan Chinese cuisine, and, for those with especially sensitive skin, almost any steaming-hot dish, have the same effect on the capillaries; they are nicknamed blushing foods.)

Underweight
This is just as undesirable as its opposite. A chronic calorie shortage may cause thinning of the subcutaneous fatty layer, making the skin look less smooth and elastic, the contours gaunt and prematurely aged. Try to maintain the weight range appropriate for your height and build.

Unbalanced and Fad Diets
Overloading on foods rich in either iodides or androgens may cause acnelike outbreaks in some susceptible people. The first category includes such foods as shellfish, seaweed, kelp, artichokes, spinach, and cabbage; the second, peanuts, organ meats, and high-gluten breads. While these items have been singled out, reactions to them are rare, far more the exception than the rule. Balance and moderation are the keys to untroubled skin. Avoid emphasizing any one food or food category to minimize the possibility of a reaction.

The Good Skin Diet:
Seven-Day Menu Plan

On this delicious, calorie-conserving plan (roughly 1,200 calories a day), you can lose weight safely and slowly at the rate of about one or two pounds a week while generously feeding your skin. If you are losing at a faster pace or wish to maintain your present weight, add a few more grains, fruits, and/or starchy vegetables or increase entrée portions slightly at lunch and dinner.

Or you might try one of these wholesome snacks each day: grated fresh fruit and a handful of golden raisins or nuts with plain yogurt; carrot sticks drizzled with a small amount of honey; apple slices peeled and parboiled in orange juice, flavored with cinnamon sticks; a small bran muffin; 2 ounces part-skim-milk cheese (Jarlsberg, Fontina, farmer) with two whole-wheat crackers or melba toast rounds; celery or endive stalks stuffed with low-fat cottage cheese and chopped chives or scallions, or dipped in herb-sprinkled plain yogurt; a thin slice of turkey or cheese wrapped around celery or lettuce. The flavorful possibilities are endless. (Both the protein and fiber in the above foods give them ample staying power, keeping you well defended against hunger pangs!)

If you are losing weight too slowly or not at all, cut back your daily intake by about 500 calories. (Buy a pocket calorie-counter book for reference.) Over a seven-day period this will add up to a saving of 3,500 calories, or the equivalent to one pound of weight. If possible, purchase a complete table of food values, listing the calorie, protein, carbohydrate, fat, vitamin and mineral content of foods, so you will be able to substitute wisely when you wish to vary the menu.

Regardless of your goals, do not skip meals. Eating three times a day is essential to the success of any healthy diet. For example, studies have repeatedly shown that missing breakfast can actually hamper efforts to lose weight by leaving you unsatisfied and causing your body to overcome the deficit later on. Nutritionally speaking, however, you never quite make up for the forsaken breakfast, no matter how well you eat during the rest of the day.

If you have no time or appetite for breakfast every morning, try to eat within at least two hours of awakening. If you are the kind of dieter who thrives best on snacking all day long instead of on three square meals, divide your portions, eating part and saving the rest for later.

Beverages at each meal should be selected from the following: decaffeinated coffee or tea, herb tea, fresh fruit or vegetable juice, bottled mineral water or seltzer (not club soda, which is too high in sodium). Skim milk is already indicated on the menu plan.

Note: Check with your physician first before following this food regimen or any other. You should also be under supervision if you stay on a reducing plan for longer than seven days.

Monday

Breakfast

> 1-egg omelet, prepared in nonstick pan, filled with 2 tablespoons low-fat cottage cheese and fresh herbs
> ½ cup assorted fresh fruit in season, topped with 1 tablespoon bran or wheat germ
> 1 slice whole-wheat toast or ½ pita bread with 1 teaspoon soft butter or margarine

Lunch

> Salad of assorted fresh vegetables (romaine, grated carrots, sliced cucumbers, green pepper, raw red cabbage, tomatoes, sprouts), garnished with slices of apple or pineapple, topped with 3 ounces farmer cheese or low-fat cottage cheese.

> Use mixture of fresh lemon juice, plain yogurt and fresh or dried herbs as dressing for vegetables, or 1 tablespoon bottled low-calorie dressing.

Dinner

½ baked cornish hen with orange slices

½ cup each steamed brussels sprouts and string beans
with 1 teaspoon soft butter or margarine

1 medium baked potato with 1 tablespoon plain yogurt, chopped fresh chives, and parsley

1 medium pear or ½ cup fresh fruit salad

Tuesday

Breakfast

⅔ cup Shredded Wheat or hot whole-grain cereal such
as Roman Meal, with ½ cup skim milk and ½
small sliced banana

Cinnamon-broiled grapefruit half (with strawberry
garnish in season)

1 small bran muffin or 1 slice whole-wheat toast
with 1 teaspoon soft butter or margarine

Lunch

3 ounces tuna, hard-cooked egg, and almond salad
(to include ½ sliced boiled egg and 1 tablespoon
slivered almonds) with 1 teaspoon mayonnaise or
1 tablespoon plain yogurt and fresh dill, served
over romaine lettuce leaves

1 slice whole-wheat bread or ½ pita bread

½ cup fresh fruit salad sprinkled with 1 tablespoon
toasted wheat germ and shredded coconut

½ cup skim milk

Dinner

4 ounces boneless chicken breast (retain skin during
baking or broiling for maximum flavor and to
prevent drying, remove skin when cooked), flavored
with fresh herbs and white wine

½ cup brown rice cooked in plain chicken broth
½ cup steamed broccoli with lemon
Spinach salad with chopped water chestnuts, sliced
   fresh mushrooms, and low-calorie or plain yogurt
   and lemon juice dressing
1 fresh apple or pear

Wednesday

Breakfast

⅔ cup hot oatmeal topped with cinnamon, 1 tablespoon raw honey or natural preserves, and 1 teaspoon toasted wheat germ
1 slice whole-wheat toast with 1 teaspoon soft butter
   or margarine
½ cup skim milk
1 cup fresh strawberries or other fruit in season

Lunch

1 slice lean meatloaf, 2 ounces lean roast beef, or 3
   ounces low-fat cheese with sprouts and romaine
   lettuce
1 slice whole-wheat bread or ½ pita bread
Salad of watercress, celery, cucumber, tomato, and
   carrots with plain yogurt and lemon juice dressing
   or 1 tablespoon low-calorie dressing
½ cup apple cider or 1 small fresh fruit

Dinner

4 ounces flounder filet baked with ¼ cup tomato
   juice, chopped fresh chives, and parsley
½ cup each steamed cauliflower and green beans
   with 1 teaspoon soft butter or margarine
1 tossed cucumber and tomato salad with 1 tablespoon low-calorie dressing
1 pear

Thursday

Breakfast

1 medium orange or ½ cup fresh-squeezed orange
  juice
1 poached egg
1 slice sprouted-wheat bread with 1 teaspoon soft
  butter or margarine
½ cup skim milk

Lunch

3 ozs. sliced fresh turkey on 1 small slice rye or pita
  bread round with 1 teaspoon mayonnaise and sprouts
  or shredded lettuce
Small salad of spinach and mixed greens, sesame
  seeds, and sliced fresh mushrooms with plain yogurt and lemon juice or 1 tablespoon low-calorie
  dressing
1 medium apple or pear
½ cup skim milk

Dinner

4 ounces broiled filet of sole with 1 teaspoon butter
  or margarine
4 ounces pasta with tomato sauce, fresh herbs, ground
  pepper, and 1 ounce freshly grated Parmesan cheese,
  or 1 baked potato with 1 tablespoon plain yogurt
  and freshly chopped chives
½ cup each steamed green beans and carrots
Small tossed green salad
½ cup fresh strawberries

Friday

Breakfast

  ½ fresh grapefruit
  1 slice rye toast spread with ¼ cup cottage cheese,
    sprinkled with cinnamon
  ½ sliced apple
  ½ cup skim milk

Lunch

  1 cup lentil soup
  3 ounces water-packed salmon, flaked, tossed with
    chopped pimiento, celery, onion, and grated car-
    rots, with 2 tablespoons plain yogurt and fresh dill
    on bed of romaine lettuce or alfalfa sprouts
  ½ cup skim milk
  1 medium pear

Dinner

  4 ounces grilled veal chops
  ½ cup brown rice or kasha
  ½ cup steamed broccoli with onions
  Small tossed salad with lemon juice
  ½ cup Mandarin orange sections

Saturday

Breakfast

  ½ fresh grapefruit
  ⅔ cup cooked Wheatena or cold whole-grain cereal
    with ½ cup skim milk, topped with 1 small sliced
    banana or 1 peach (fresh or canned without syrup),
    plus 1 tablespoon toasted wheat germ or bran

Lunch

½ cup baked macaroni and cheese casserole
Fresh coleslaw with 1 teaspoon mayonnaise, or tossed
  salad of romaine, green pepper, tomato, cucumber, raw cauliflower, lemon juice, assorted spices
1 apple
½ cup skim milk

Dinner

¼ roasted chicken basted with a small amount of
  olive oil, white wine, and fresh herbs (e.g., rose-
  mary, tarragon)
½ medium baked acorn squash
½ cup steamed Chinese cabbage
Spinach and sliced mushroom salad with lemon juice
½ cup fresh strawberries or salad of fresh fruits in
  season

Sunday

Breakfast

1 slice whole-wheat French toast
½ cantaloupe filled with sliced fresh strawberries
½ cup skim milk

Lunch

4 ounces curried chicken or tuna salad (4 ounces
  cooked, diced skinless chicken or white meat tuna
  with ½ tablespoon plain yogurt, 1 teaspoon curry
  powder, ¼ cup drained crushed pineapple, chopped
  celery and onion, apple chunks, shredded cocoa-
  nut, and a few raisins, blended well and tossed
  over bed of alfalfa sprouts, spinach, or romaine
  leaves)

1 small bran muffin
½ cup skim milk

Dinner

4 ounces vegetable and brown rice casserole topped
  with 2 ounces Monterey Jack cheese
½ cup each steamed carrots and zucchini with 1
  teaspoon melted butter or margarine
Small tossed salad with sliced green pepper
Small bunch grapes (about 15)

CHAPTER 12

YOUR SKIN DIRECTORY: AFFLICTIONS MINOR TO MAJOR

No matter how vigilant you are, human skin is not always predictable, nor does it necessarily remain picture-perfect. It is prey to a host of minor lumps, bumps, blotches, specks, and other imperfections, which might well be called "the little uglies."

According to a recent report by the U.S. Department of Health, Education and Welfare, more than twenty-five million Americans suffer from at least one skin disorder, a number that remains relatively constant from year to year. Many of the complaints are of unknown origin. Others are associated with heredity, allergy, irregularities in metabolism, underlying disease, or chronic injury. Some, such as psoriasis and eczema, are noninfectious; others are caused by bacteria or fungi and can spread from one part of the body to another or from person to person.

Paradoxically, some of the least troublesome skin problems medically can be among the most annoying or embarrassing. The common wart and mole are notorious examples. Happily, however, most uglies are easily treated. With modern know-how and some old-fashioned motivation, chances are good that whatever minor affliction ails you can be quickly, painlessly, and inexpensively done away with. And recent breakthroughs in treatment promise to eradicate the major ones, too.

Moles

Moles are technically tumors of the skin, bits of extra-pigmented tissue that range in color from flesh-colored to brown, black, or bluish black. Some are raised, hairy, or sandpaper-rough in texture, while others are flat and smooth. Depending on their size and location, which can be any-where on the skin, and whether single or in clusters, moles can be decidedly unflattering or else attractive beauty marks. Generally they appear during the first two decades of life, though some may make their debut around the age of forty.

Moles may turn lighter or darker or fade away com-pletely with time, or grow larger and more conspicuous during puberty and pregnancy. Some become raised above skin level enough for them to develop a small stalk and eventually fall off by themselves. Exactly what causes them is not yet known, but the vast majority of these growths are benign. Even so, you should see a doctor immediately if you notice any change. An alteration in size, shape, color, texture, sensitivity or the presence of pain, irritation, discharge, bleeding, or itching could indi-cate malignancy. *Note:* Congenital moles have a greater chance of turning cancerous than those that appear later on. For this reason, it's advisable to have them removed as early in life as possible—just to play it safe.

Moles can be safely and easily removed by shaving them off just at the skin surface and destroying the base with an electric needle or by excising them surgically. These are relatively quick, painless procedures that can be performed in a physician's office. Some slight scarring is a possibility, so if you want one removed for purely cosmetic reasons, consider whether you might be trading in one blemish for another. Scarring can be minimized if your dermatologist works within natural skin folds and applies sutures correctly.

Bandages can be removed within hours of surgery or not used at all, since air helps dry tissue and speed healing. Normally a tiny scab will form and then fall away within a week or two. Within four to eight weeks the skin should be completely cleared, though the resulting scar may continue to fade over a period of months. An antibiotic ointment applied two to three times a day can soften skin, aid healing, and minimize crusting or scab formation. Hairs growing out of moles should not be removed by electrolysis, or else the surface may become over-irritated.

Warts

While rarely serious, warts can be among the most maddeningly stubborn and unpredictable disorders of all. Some resist outright drastic means of removal, including burning, cutting, and caustic solutions. Others disappear spontaneously or may be hypnotized away in days by a local mystic!

Warts are another variety of benign tumor, but unlike moles, almost never become malignant. And we do know where they come from: a common virus, which enters the skin, often through a cut or scrape, and infects the upper layers of the epidermis. If you shave, scratch, or pick them, warts can spread easily from fingers, hands, face, back, or soles of feet to anywhere on the body or even be passed on to someone else. Since the majority eventually vanish on their own, the only reason to remove them is if they are painful or unsightly. Warts can be raised or flat or only slightly elevated, smooth or rough, grayish brown or flesh-colored, and range from pinhead and lentil size to very large growths. Among the various major types are the following.

Common Warts

The hands, fingers, and knees are the usual targets for this variety, which consists of rough-textured, clearly defined, and generally painless eruptions. Freshly formed lesions are skin-colored, turning yellowish tan and coarser with age. A typical pattern is a central or mother wart surrounded by a cluster of satellites or offspring, which often arise after isolated warts have been picked and manipulated.

Flat Warts

These flesh- or tan-colored spots commonly appear around the face, neck, chest, and hands. In men they are often spread by shaving very closely.

Filiform Warts

These project from an often pale-pink base (generally over face, neck, eyelids, and lips) and have pointed, delicate, often hardened tips.

Plantar Warts

Probably the most tenacious and hardest to treat, this type roots itself on the feet, usually on weight-bearing areas (soles and heels). Firm, flat, or slightly elevated, these are often driven deeply into the skin by walking, and cause great pain and tenderness. If they occur bilaterally—on both feet simultaneously—walking may be all but impossible.

Initially the plantar wart appears as a single small dot. Often mistaken for a splinter, it is poked and picked at, which only causes it to enlarge. Ultimately it may assume a mosaic pattern consisting of scores of small adjacent growths or else may be large, singular, and several inches across. Unlike a callus, this wart is usually not crisscrossed by normal ridges of the skin, and this is one way of identifying it.

Perilungual Warts
Nail-biting may result in a tumor near the nail or in the folds, affecting several fingers and, less commonly, the toes. If this variety grows below the nail surface, it can end up penetrating as deeply as a plantar wart. Pain may be considerable, since the pressure of the wart often displaces the nail.

Genital Warts
Also known as moist or veneral warts (the medical term is condyloma acuminata), these cauliflower- or raspberry-shaped growths occur most commonly in the ano-genital area and range from fleshy-pink to gray. The only type of wart that has the potential to turn malignant if not treated early is a genital variety that can erupt in people over forty. Called the Buschke-Lowenstein giant condyloma, it may grow up to two inches long.

Treatment: Your Choice
For those who do not simply want to watch warts disappear, dermatologists and other physicians have a number of promising, though not yet foolproof, methods of removing them.

Cryotherapy freezes warts away. In this treatment, liquid nitrogen at a temperature of $-196°C$ is applied to the wart for fifteen to thirty seconds. The ultra-freezing induces the formation of blisters which disturbs the environment of the virus-infected cells yet leaves the "basement" membrane intact. The advantages are little or no scarring and no need of local anesthesia. However, a subtle throbbing or burning sensation may accompany treatment, and the area may remain sensitive for several days. Larger warts may require several cryotherapy sessions for complete removal.

Curettage involves lifting out the entire wart with a razor-sharp instrument, then carefully scraping the edges to prevent viral particles from taking root again.

Electrodesiccation employs a short burst of high-frequency electric current (delivered with a fine-tipped needle) to destroy infected cells. The procedure requires an injection of an anesthetic into the surrounding skin. A small crust or scab develops, followed by some scarring, which usually appears less conspicuous with time.

Chemosurgery destroys infected cells with topical applications of an acid such as trichloracetic or salicyclic acid, phenol or silver nitrate, or the phenol-nitric acid-salicylic acid paste method. Vitamin A acid (retinoic acid) can successfully peel away scattered small, flat facial warts.

For plantar and other large warts, a solution of formalin brushed on with a cotton-tipped applicator is a reliable alternative to painful surgery. The physician covers the formalin-treated wart with a salicylic acid plaster tape. The patch is removed, along with layers of dead skin, then reapplied. This method, which may also involve local applications of trichloracetic acid, makes the tissue easier to remove.

For do-it-yourselfers, Compound W and other drugstore remedies may also be quite effective for certain growths. In using these, follow label instructions carefully and plan on at least a month of daily treatment before seeing results.

What about the thousands of bizarre nostrums and folk remedies? Do they really work? Consider a few popular old wives' tales: a copper penny, a slice of raw potato, half an apple, a length of yarn knotted with the number of warts on your skin. Other approaches include prayer and hypnotism. What they may all have in common is a belief by the user that they will work. Hypnotic suggestion, faith healing, and strong, positive thinking (autosuggestion or self-hypnosis) can all stop blood flow to a wart, thereby starving it and causing it to dry out and disappear. This has led many doctors to suspect a body/mind connection in the origin of warts, possibly involving stress and the resulting immune response. Of course, since most warts clear up spontaneously anyway, the folk remedies—or rather the conviction that they cure—may just be a happy coincidence, after all!

Though a number of methods can be successful, however, no method will necessarily work at any given time or ensure lasting results. Warts are curiously unpredictable, so several approaches may have to be tried and tested before any visible improvement is seen. No physician, however brilliant or diligent, can guarantee the wart(s) will never return.

What's new and on the horizon in treating warts? Today the most resistant growths can be snuffed out with a carbon dioxide laser used at very low power, an expensive, high-tech option that may be considered if other methods fail. However, this treatment is not foolproof.

DNCB, a potent sensitizer, is now also being used as a last-resort method for hard-to-treat cases. DNCB may leave behind a severe poison ivy-like rash in place of the original wart. In one recent study, injection of a mumps skin test antigen (vaccine) into a single wart eliminated that wart and caused all the other warts on the body to disappear as well. Thirty-five people with multiple resistant or plantar warts were treated, and almost three-quarters of them experienced complete clearing; all had formerly failed to respond to liquid nitrogen, radiation, excision, and electrodesiccation. (Those who had not had a case of the mumps or the mumps vaccine were immunized before treatment.) If the warts did not shrink by the sixth week, a second injection was made. This apparently safe, inexpensive, and nonscarring method is believed to work by triggering a natural immune response in the body.

A drug called Blenoxane (bleomycin sulfate) is another effective and safe treatment for resistant plantar warts. Also a simple procedure, this requires no anesthesia, electrodesiccation or protective dressing. Moreover, it is inexpensive, well tolerated, and leaves no scar. A group of thirty-six patients ranging in age from four to sixty-eight were treated with bleomycin. Eight out of ten patients with a single wart, seven out of nine with two or three warts, and twelve out of seventeen with multiple warts were cured after one or two courses of therapy. The warts did not recur within three months after treatment.

Atopic Dermatitis

Atopic dermatitis is a hereditary disease that occurs in both infants and adults. If persistent, the often intolerably itchy, potentially disfiguring inflammation can be emotionally crippling. While the condition usually clears by the age of thirty, occasionally it can linger throughout life, leading sufferers to seek some desperate solutions.

The disease typically runs in families along with susceptibility to asthma, hay fever, and other allergic disorders. In babies, atopic dermatitis is often referred to as infantile eczema and is centered chiefly on the face, scalp, neck, and diaper areas. When the child frantically scratches and rubs the dry, cracked skin with his hands or any object within reach for relief, he only succeeds in spreading, irritating, and possibly infecting the condition. If it becomes severely inflamed, the skin starts to ooze and crust. In over half the children affected, the disease disappears spontaneously between the ages of two and four, though it may recur in early adulthood. (In the other half, the infantile disorder progresses directly into the adult form.)

Beyond infancy, atopic dermatitis commonly finds its way to the bends of elbows and knees, the scalp, face, neck, upper back, chest, and shoulders, arms, fingers, palms, feet, and even the genital area. Hay fever or asthma may sometimes precede or accompany the symptoms at this stage. The problem worsens in winter when interiors are dry and the skin is exposed to hot baths and chafing wool. Vigorous scratching or rubbing wears away the fragile, already sensitive tissues, induces bleeding, and leaves the affected areas more prone to infection. It also releases fluids, which eventually dry out and form a crusty covering on the surface. Even when left untouched, intermittent flares and remissions are characteristic of the disease. In a flare, the itching, swelling, and redness intensify and the dermatitis spreads; in a remission, symptoms subside and even disappear.

Emotional turmoil can be both a consequence and a cause of the disorder. Psychiatric studies have shown that victims experience a mixture of disturbing, self-destructive feelings, among them a sense of worthlessness, despair, extreme depression, repressed hostility, and heightened sensitivity. Both physicians and patients alike acknowledge that the unremitting, inescapable suffering can trigger profound personality changes. Chronic personal stress, in turn, can aggravate the condition and sabotage treatment.

Aside from a strongly suspected genetic link, the causes of atopic dermatitis remain elusive. Along with emotional upsets, seasonal changes, contact with irritants such as rough, chafing wool and harsh soaps or detergents, cutting oils and greases, dusts and airborne allergens, and overly strenuous activity can intensify a predisposition or an already existing case in both children and adults.

The primary aim of treatment is to soothe the inflammation and curb the itching sensation so that the skin can start to heal itself (and so that no further damage will be inflicted by scratching). Another strategy is to fend off any bacteria that have invaded the sensitive tissues. Of course, if a specific environmental agent is believed responsible—paints, cleaning products, aerosol sprays—isolating, identifying, and eliminating it are essential for lasting results. Keeping sweating to a minimum and avoiding abrupt extremes of temperature, coarse, excessive, or ill-fitting clothing, heavy cosmetic lotions, and rigorous exercise are also advised.

Compresses of ice-water, milk, or Burow's solution (available in drugstores), patted on repeatedly for ten minutes at intervals throughout the day can ease crusted, irritated lesions. Antihistamine pills, tar-based preparations, and tepid oatmeal soaks added to the bath can all help quiet affected areas, reduce swelling, and accelerate drying. Oral antibiotics can be used to control secondary infection; your physician should do a culture to determine the bacterial source so that he can prescribe the appropriate medication. Under a doctor's watchful eye, steroid creams are another potent remedy, best applied after a shower or bath, then covered tightly in some cases with a clear but non-breathing plastic such as Saran Wrap. Long-term use of steroid preparations should be avoided unless specifically prescribed. (Minimal doses of oral steroids for the briefest time necessary may work wonders in difficult cases.)

Tepid oatmeal or cornstarch baths are naturally soothing, as is plain water splashed with dispersible bath oil. While petroleum jelly is neutral on most atopic skin, some patients do not tolerate any greases well. For them, a jellylike emulsion such as Cetaphil lotion is a good emollient, and soap substitutes like Lowila should be considered.

To encourage healing and pamper skin, wear soft, light cotton clothes whenever possible and keep play, work, and sleep areas cool and well ventilated. Take sponge baths daily and avoid hot, soapy showers.

When the condition resists treatment, it may be best to limit or avoid potentially troublesome foods such as cow's milk, peanuts, wheat products, and eggs for at least a few weeks on a trial basis. Occasionally objects such as feather dusters, pillows, comforters and mattresses, carpets, drapes, certain toys, pets, garments, and furs may also cause a flareup. In some cases a change of environment, preferably to a warm, arid climate, offers dramatic relief.

Steer clear of vaccines, since atopic skin is very susceptible to infection by certain viruses (especially the herpes simplex or cold sore variety). The disorder also leaves its victims more susceptible to severe reactions to penicillin, foreign blood serum, and other drugs. For this reason, avoid exposure to such agents unless they are essential either to prevent or to treat a serious condition.

Contact Dermatitis

This common complaint is caused by direct exposure to an irritating substance. Hair follicles, sweat glands, and cracks in the skin caused by dryness can all be inviting entryways for chemicals at home or work.

Irritant Reactions
Skin directly exposed to harsh chemicals and other harmful agents can react in a variety of ways. If the offending materials (called primary irritants) touch the skin in the right concentrations for a long enough time they will result in a condition called *contact* dermatitis—and even one-time exposure may be sufficient. Primary irritants such as

acid, alkali, ammonia, strong soaps, and detergents can inflame the outer layers of anybody's skin. Some irritants produce no visible change or pain on initial contact, but they do break down the skin's defenses.

Less commonly, other substances, such as leather and rubber—which cause no trouble for most of us—may give rise to a similar flareup only after a certain "incubation period" when the skin becomes sensitive or allergic to the material. At this point, any further, even casual, exposure will produce an eruption of the skin known as allergic contact dermatitis. (The agent responsible is called a contactant.)

How the allergy "happens": First you make contact with a substance; then changes occur in the skin which make it highly susceptible to that same substance if it is touched again—anywhere from weeks to decades later. In fact, some people who have been repeatedly exposed to an agent for many years will suddenly experience an allergic reaction to it for no apparent reason. That means all contactants, familiar and brand new, are under suspicion as possible causes of allergic contact dermatitis until proven innocent. Also, a given chemical can act as both an allergic sensitizer and a primary irritant.

Regardless of the cause, most cases of contact dermatitis look and feel alike: with itching, reddening, swelling papules, and tiny eruptions or blisters called vessicles which form crusts and scales when they break. (The size and shape of the eruption depend on where the contactant has touched the skin.) As reported in *The Manual Of Contact Dermatitis*, by Sigfrid Fregert (Yearbook Medical Publishers, Copenhagen, 1974), if left untreated, the condition can eventually become chronic and the skin may turn dark, leathery, and cracked. "Allergic contact dermatitis is difficult to distinguish from many forms of eczema and rashes brought on by systemic reactions and bacterial or fungal infections, as well as those caused by primary irritants," the author points out.

A patch test is a quick, reliable test for allergy: For

example, one woman complained of dermatitis on the mouth and her doctor naturally suspected her favorite brand of lipstick. However, since her condition persisted even after she stopped using the product, he investigated further with a patch test. This involves applying a small amount and appropriate concentration of a suspected substance to the gauze part of an adhesive and leaving it on the skin for a fixed period. After it's removed the area is observed for any reaction. The culprit turned out to be the nickel coating on her hairpins which she had repeatedly placed in her mouth as she styled her hair every night.

Remember, while almost anybody can suffer a skin irritation, relatively few people have allergic reactions. (Poison ivy is a notable exception as most of us are highly sensitive to the oleoresins in the plant.) But there is no sure way to predict whether someone will become allergic to anything. Doctors do know that nickel, rubber, dyes (especially the permanent kind), and chromates (found in leather, bleaches, paints, and glues) are among the agents most likely to induce an allergic contact dermatitis.

Hand Eczema

To get more specific, the most distressing dermatitis of all is the one that affects your hands. The problem is equally frustrating for the dermatologist since hand eczemas of entirely different causes may closely resemble each other. Allergies to materials that contact your hands or irritation from soap, water, and detergents may produce a dermatitis which is hard to distinguish from atopic eczema, psoriasis, nummular eczema, and fungus or yeast infections.

Many cases of hand eczema involve a number of causes, as the list details below. Secondary infections, irritation, allergy and trauma may all be playing a role by the time a patient reaches a doctor.

Housewives' eczema: caused by exposure to drying, degreasing and irritating agents in contact with hands.

Allergic contact dermatitis: caused by a specific agent or chemical; a patch test can pinpoint the source. (See above.)

Psoriasis: usually accompanied by psoriasis on the nails and a family history of the disease.

Atopic hand eczema: occurs in those with a personal or family history of eczema, asthma or hay fever; similar to housewives' eczema. Specific irritants are common sources and emotional upset may also trigger a sudden outbreak.

Dishydrotic eczema: groups of deep-seated small blisters which itch intensely may suddenly appear on the sides of fingers and palms especially, and some people with this type rash perspire excessively on both the palms and soles, often in response to emotional turmoil.

Pustular bacterid: a rare type of hand eczema consisting of blisters and pustules on fingers and palms, probably in response to internal infection.

Fungus, bacterial, or yeast infections: on the hands, may be diagnosed by doing a culture (smear of pus or scraping of scales) and looking under a microscope for the organisms.

Id reactions: probably allergic rashes on the hands coming from materials absorbed from the feet that are infected with bacteria or fungi, or otherwise inflamed.

Nummular eczema: shows up as round, red, scaling, crusting or blistering areas usually on the backs of the hands. May occur in those with excessively dry skin, a history of allergies, or for no apparent reason at all.

Treatment

Cleansers, detergents, and many other irritants strip away protective surface oils and undermine the skin's capacity to retain water. Moisture within the outer layers of skin is in large measure what keeps it feeling soft and smooth. Without lubricating water and oils, skin is more susceptible to rashes and itching.

The aim of treatment is to:

1. avoid irritants and allergens
2. put water back into the skin and seal it in with a cream or oil
3. relieve the itching
4. clear up the rash with cortisone creams, tar lotions, etc.

Usually creams rubbed on pre-dampened skin alone are effective. Sometimes, however, internal medicines are necessary to clear the rash. For continual protection, use either dermal gloves (made of thin white cotton, also known as pallbearer gloves) when handling dry, irritating substances or cotton-lined rubber gloves (Bluettes, for example) when handling wet or moist ones. Avoid direct contact with:

detergents, bathroom cleansers
solvents
hot water
alcohol
urine in diaper pails
paints, paint thinners
rough cloths
bleaches
lacquers
hair preparations (including shampoos, dyes, permanent wave solutions)
chalk
floor, furniture, or car polishes
gasoline, lighter fluid
garlic
potatoes
okra
citrus fruits

raw meats
vegetables
onions

Ideally, your hands should not stay in gloves for longer than half an hour at a time, since perspiration also can aggravate dermatitis. When your hands must be immersed in water for household chores, cotton gloves (sprinkle powder inside them) under lined rubber gloves will absorb excess moisture from sweating. This combination is best for doing dishes, sorting or changing diapers, washing bathrooms, cleaning sinks, scrubbing floors, peeling raw vegetables, mixing drinks, handling raw meats, etc. If water is spilled over the cuffs of the gloves, remove immediately and replace with another pair.

If wet work cannot be avoided, try to do it all at once rather than put your hands in and out of water. After you finish, soak hands in clean, cool water for about five minutes, then rub a cortisone or hand cream into the wet skin. Pat dry, then reapply the cream.

Do not use any medicines, soaps, or hand creams without your doctor's approval.

Use a soap substitute such as Dove, Phase III, or Alpha Keri Soap. You may also try other mild soaps or soap substitutes such as Lowila, Basis, Emulave, Neutrogena, Oilatum, or Kauma.

Avoid very hot water, even with your gloves on.

Don't apply excessive pressure on the hands or rub them vigorously.

If itching occurs, immerse hands in cold water to which some bath oil has been added. Follow with a thin film of cortisone cream. As for bath oils, choose Alpha Keri, Lubath, Mapo, Nutraspa, Aveeno, Domol, Balnetar, Kauma, and similar products.

After your hands appear normal, continue applying cortisone cream on a gradually decreasing basis for the next four to six weeks. Even though your hands may appear trouble-free, they are still quite sensitive for some time after the rash clears and they demand not only continued avoidance of irritants but also continued treatment.

If you expose your hands to an irritating substance, even water, after the rash has cleared and you have discontinued treatment, prevent problems by applying a hand cream such as Keri Cream, Nutroderm, Carmol Cream, Nivea, Eucerin, Neutrogena, Lubriderm, and Aqua-care HP.

Atopic Dermatitis or Eczema Questionnaire
These questions will help you pinpoint the source of your skin condition and help your doctor prescribe the best treatment.

Circle or Answer:
Does anyone in your family have eczema, asthma, hay fever?

Do you suffer from any allergies, hay fever, asthma?

Do you break out on the skin?
    Where?
    What does eruption look like? Is it scaly, blistered, red, swollen?

Is your skin dry?

How many times a week do you shower or bathe?
    Do you use hot, tepid, or cool water?
    Bubble bath?
    Bath oil? Type?
    What soap? Type?
    Do you rub dry or pat dry?

Do you use a moisturizer?
    Where?
    Name?
    When?

Do you use a sauna or swim?

Do you use a fabric softener? Name?

Does eating any foods make you itch, break out, or get hives? Cow's milk, eggs, fish, wheat, peanuts, chocolates? Any other foods?

Do you itch more around or with:
    Summer, winter, spring, fall?
    Dogs, cats, birds, other household pets?
    Wool, nylon fur, other fabrics?
    Dust?
    Smoke?
    Foods: eggs, fish, wheat, peanuts, other?

Do you have any animals at home? What kinds?

Do lanolin-containing creams make you itch?

Does perspiration make you itch more? What sports make your skin look worse?

Is there a climate that seems to help you more? Warm and dry? Warm and moist? Other?

Is your condition aggravated when you have an infection, cold, bronchitis, kidney infection?

Do you get frequent skin infections?

What are you using on your skin now? (Indicate types or names of products used.)
    Lotions?
    Soap?
    Medicines?

What pills or shots are you taking now?

Are you receiving allergy injections now, or have you had them in the past?

What medications have helped in the past?

Have you had fever blisters? Are they usually widespread?

Have you been vaccinated? Did you have any reactions to the vaccination?

Have you ever been tested for allergies?
    Scratch or prick test?
    Patch tests?
    What were the results?

Are you allergic to anything? Perfume? Soap? Nickel? Jewelry? Other?

Are you allergic to any medications? Aspirin? Penicillin? Sulfa drugs? Other?

Poison Ivy

When you see three leaves and a shiny surface, watch out! Or, as the familiar saying goes, "Leaflets three, let it be!" The notorious "poisons," ivy, oak, and sumac, are probably the most common cause of allergic contact dermatitis in the United States. While the rash is usually triggered by direct contact with the plants' oily compounds (called catechols), you can also pick it up by wearing clothes contaminated with the offending chemicals. All parts of the plant are poisonous, including roots and bare stems, and can work their damage as easily in winter as in summer.

Misnamed a poison, the plant is actually an allergen—capable of inducing an allergic reaction after future exposure to it. When an allergic change results from exposure to poison ivy, a skin inflammation (dermatitis) occurs at the point of contact with any part of the plant. The first time skin is exposed, usually no reaction will occur. As reported in the pamphlet, "Poison Plant Rashes," prepared by the American Medical Association and The American Academy of Dermatology, if either a first-time or later encounter initiates the allergic state the dermatitis will appear in roughly seven to fourteen days. All future exposures will then trigger dermatitis within a few hours or usually up to about two to five days later.

A good number of those who consider themselves "immune" to poison ivy probaby have had either very subtle reactions or a low degree of allergic sensitivity to the plant, or else they have had little or no significant contact. No one can ever be certain of being or remaining insensitive to poison ivy and all precautions should be taken to avoid exposure, regardless of a previous "unblemished" record.

The eruptions caused by poison ivy, oak, and sumac look identical: The typically reddening, blistering, itching rash often breaks out in short, straight-line streaks, caused by the leaf tips' brushing against your skin as you walk past the plant. The extent of the outbreak depends on the amount of catechols deposited on the skin and your level of reactivity.

Contrary to myth, neither the redness nor the blister fluid can cause the rash to spread, nor can cleansing with soap and water. In fact, always wash as thoroughly and quickly as possible after contact to help flush away the oily compounds. The condition only *appears* to spread because of differences in the time the lesions appear. (Areas in greatest contact with the plant will react the earliest, giving the misleading impression that any late-erupting lesions have resulted from a spread of the earlier ones.) Blisters can occasionally be invaded by bacteria and the resulting pustular infection may then extend to other areas of skin.

There are a number of ways to "catch" poison ivy— and that means you will not necessarily know if you have been exposed. Recently, for example, a man came in for treatment who had contracted it when he changed a tire on his car that had run over the plant several hours before. Another possible source of contamination is the family pet. Dogs and cats brush against the plants and then are petted by unsuspecting owners. Clothing and other objects are potential carriers, since they can retain the penetrating poison resins for months after contact. Interestingly, ivy is chemically related to the cashew, mango, Indian marking nut tree (source of India ink), and Japanese lacquer tree. So contact with any of these or their products could also bring on the rash if you have previously been exposed to the plant.

The itching and inflammation typical of poison ivy is the result of a defense reaction by your body's immune system. This explains why many people with asthma do not break out in the rash; their immune systems are impaired and no longer react to the catechols.

Treatment

If you know you have been exposed to the plant or its resins, shower thoroughly and immediately; you have about an hour to wash off the oils before they have a chance to penetrate the skin surface and produce the rash. Clean thoroughly under the fingernails. If the itching has already begun and you have come down with a mild case, compresses of clean cotton cloths soaked in Burow's solution (aluminum sulfate and calcium acetate) will offer prompt relief as will pads soaked in milk, ice, or salt water, calamine lotion, and creams. A mild oral antihistamine can be administered to relieve itching and discomfort. A tepid bath will reduce inflammation if eruptions are widespread. Treat clothing like your skin; wash it immediately. Never burn the leaves of poison ivy or any irritating plant, since this will only release the potent resins via fumes and smoke, inviting a far more serious and widespread reaction. If swelling or blistery eruptions occur around the eyes, apply compresses of diluted boric acid or salt water (1 teaspoon salt to 1 pint of tepid water.) Over-the-counter hydrocortisone preparations give very little relief for other than very mild cases. Your doctor may prescribe topical and/or systemic corticosteroids for more severe outbreaks.

While extremely rare, a serious enough case can give rise to skin infection. If the rash lingers too long or appears too near the eyes or other sensitive areas, it is advisable to see your physician.

Body Rashes

Aside from irritations triggered by local contact, these may be allergic reactions or warning signals—symptoms of underlying illness. If any rash starts oozing, smelling, itching excessively, or turning worse after treatment, see a doctor immediately. For mild cases, baking soda or oatmeal (Aveeno powder) added to bath water or the cooling resin from the aloe plant—released by simply breaking off the tip of one of the leaves—applied directly to troubled skin, along with the remedies cited above for atopic or allergic contact dermatitis are all reliable soothers.

Heat Rash

Heat rash, characterized by slightly raised red bumps, is caused by perspiration trapped under tightly woven clothing in a hot, humid environment, especially during strenuous exercise. Favorite sites are the front and sides of the chest, under the breasts, and the bend in elbows and knees. Wearing natural, loose, lightweight clothing, dusting frequently with powder, and moving to cooler surroundings indoors whenever possible may prevent or minimize the problem.

Sweating can also cause rash-forming chemicals to leach out from costume jewelry onto your skin. Covering nickel or platinum-coated accessories with clear nail polish may prevent the leaching effect.

Hives (Urticaria)

These itching, stinging, often painful welts are actually symptoms rather than a disorder in themselves. The chronic, lingering kind may signal the presence of an underlying infection, while a sudden, short-lived flareup is the body's response to an allergen—an offending food or drug, extremes of temperature, an emotional outburst, or even exposure to the sun.

Hives themselves are caused by a leakage of blood serum from blood vessels into the skin. This happens when an irritant or stimulant activates sensitive tissues (specialized mast cells located beneath the skin) to produce a chemical called histamine. Histamine is released during certain conditions, and the amount and circumstances vary according to a person's sensitivity. For those who are exquisitely responsive, for example, heat or cold or even the subtlest pressure is sufficient for the histamine reaction. In other cases, the mast cells respond to changes in the levels of hormones and other internal chemicals that may be brought about by overexertion or emotional stress.

Approximately fifteen to twenty percent of the population experience at least one episode of urticaria during their lifetime. At first the weals are red, but because they contain fluid, they become white as the skin stretches over them. After eighteen hours or so, they subside and usually vanish without a trace, though they may spread occasionally.

Interestingly, physicians have noted an underlying emotional profile shared by many urticaria patients. Feelings of helplessness, anxiety, and suppressed rage are typical, for example. People who are otherwise active and energetic may feel trapped, passive, unable to mobilize their energies in the face of conflict. Hives are a possible psychosomatic reaction, a physical manifestation of this emotional state.

Simple hives are also commonly associated with eating an unusual food, such as a dish of strawberries or a deliciously deviled crab. They arise almost every time such foods are eaten, especially if alcoholic beverages accompany the meal. A wide range of other edibles may be responsible, among them, citrus fruits, shellfish, wheat products, chocolate, eggs, nuts, bananas, milk, tomatoes, navy beans, mushrooms, cabbage, pickles, onions, garlic, grapes, pineapple, fresh pork, ginger, pepper and other spices, curried dishes, coffee, and tea. The salicylate family, which includes aspirin, wintergreen, root beer, sarsaparilla, and mint flavorings are also common suspects.

Still other offenders may include menthol-containing products such as throat lozenges, cigarettes, and shaving creams. Substances used in cosmetics, hand lotions, contraceptives, gargles, and scalp applications, chemical preservatives, food dyes, and penicillin, along with allergy to molds, dust, pollen, plants, insects, and animal dander can activate hives as well. Infections such as dental abscesses, tonsilitis, sinusitis, cystitis, and ringworm occasionally cause them, too. Part of your treatment is to keep an accurate record of the foods you eat and the medications you take, the time and occasion when you break out, and how long the reaction lasts—all to help isolate the source of trouble.

If hives persist or flare up frequently over a period of several months (chronic urticaria), you should have a thorough examination, including blood and urine tests, a chest X ray, perhaps dental X rays and a sinus check. The key to controlling hives, acute or chronic, is to get to the bottom of them, literally. Sometimes, of course, no apparent cause is found and hives still flourish even if living or eating habits are radically changed. (Likewise, they often disappear while conditions remain the same.)

In any case, the goal is to reduce itching and discomfort with topical mild lotions such as Aladerm or Nutraderm, along with cool or warm showers, soothing baths, ice packs, and witch hazel rubs. Oral antihistamines can also keep hives at bay and minimize recurrence. Aspirin and hot showers should be avoided, since these tend to aggravate the condition in some people. Remember, you cannot give hives to anyone else, and the problem is rarely hazardous to health. Medical attention is necessary, however, if large, internal swellings that threaten to impair breathing occur in the area of the mouth and throat or if the face itself swells, particularly around the lips and eyes.

Hives are not easy to treat: Don't be surprised if your doctor has to engage in some time-consuming trial and error to find out the proper combination or dosage of antihistamine medications that will help you. But while the itching may seem unbearable for a while, the condition ultimately does respond to treatment—all that's required is considerable patience and persistence by both you and your physician.

Note: People with a personal or family history of asthma, hay fever, or migraine headache seem more susceptible than average to stubborn, chronic hives.

Pruritus (Itching Disorders)

A variety of skin diseases are believed to liberate protein-dissolving enzymes that irritate the nerve endings responsible for sensing heat, cold, and pain. These disturbed nerve endings, in turn, produce itching as a result of erratic signals sent to the brain. Since the same nerve network is involved in both itch and pain, many drugs that quell pain or temporarily numb the skin will also relieve itching.

While scratching is the natural, instinctive way to relieve an itch, it can also damage the skin, leave lasting scars, spread an existing rash, and aggravate the itch or pain. However, scratching or pricking the skin some distance away from a rash, bite, or weal can offer temporary relief. It stimulates an area of skin served by the same nerves as those producing the itch, thus blocking or diverting the original sensation.

Prime among the itching skin disorders are:

Lichens simplex chronicus
Also sometimes called localized neurodermatitis, this syndrome can be caused by an insect bite, a chafing collar, repeated scratching of an area of skin, stress, anxiety, or underlying disease. The back of the neck and limbs are common sites, though it can occur anywhere. Lichenification—a thickening of the skin with marked surface lines and discolored, dry, close-set bumps—results from continual rubbing and scratching. The coarsened skin is acutely

sensitive to further itching, setting up a vicious cycle.

Treatment involves curbing the itch with steroid creams, ointments, or gels or a tape impregnated with steroid (codran tape). These should be covered tightly with plastic and changed daily. Sometimes physicians use heavy bandages soaked with gelatin and zinc oxide to reduce itching. Injections of diluted steroids into the affected skin may also be helpful in stubborn cases.

Xerosis

Xerosis is another name for scaly, dried-out skin. When vigorously scratched, it can react with swelling, oozing, or crusted patches, similar to those of eczema. Frequent hot showers, harsh soaps, saunas, and steambaths all play a role in stripping the skin of moisture. As oil gland activity declines with age, surface fluids evaporate more readily, also setting the stage for dryness. During winter, over-heated rooms and low outdoor humidity further aggravate the condition.

Treating xerosis is a relatively simple matter. Shower briefly in tepid water or immerse yourself in baths for no longer than five to ten minutes, using a mild soap suitable for very dry or sensitive skin (see Chapter 9). While skin is still slightly damp after superficial towel-drying, apply a moisturizer, preferably a cream-based one such as Nivea. Sometimes a steroid ointment can be used for a short period of time to reduce itching and inflammation. Humidify rooms properly, avoid harsh detergents, and wear cotton-lined rubber gloves while working for any extended time in water (for example, while doing the dishes or washing the car).

Psychosomatic itching

As mentioned earlier, itching can be one manifestation of emotional distress. The complaint itself may be widespread or localized and is usually most intense in the evening.

Sufferers scratch endlessly, picking away at their skin and often inflicting considerable damage in the process. Psychotherapy can help call attention to the problem. Once a person recognizes that the condition is emotionally based rather than rooted in any organic, bodily disturbance, he or she can begin to heal by resolving the underlying conflict. Doctors may prescribe antidepressants for a short period to help speed recovery. Cool compresses, baths with powdered oatmeal or baking soda, and topical steroid creams or lotions containing menthol or phenol can offer local relief and help keep the patient's mind away from his or her skin.

Itching: Guidelines for Relief

Scabies, shingles, eczema, atopic dermatitis, and allergic rashes, among other skin plagues, are often accompanied by intense itching. For general relief, a host of over-the-counter products are available today. These include skin-soothing, cooling, absorbent ingredients such as calamine; numbing or freezing agents (anesthetics) such as benzocaine, which temporarily block the itching and burning sensations; and pain-relievers (analgesics) such as menthol. If your problem gets worse, discontinue all medication and see your doctor. Oral antihistamines such as Benadryl help prevent histamine, the irritating body chemical, from reaching and swelling skin cells.

One recent answer to chronic, rash-related itching is a lotion derived from drugs commonly prescribed to treat depression (called tricyclics). Considered more effective than traditional topical steroid drugs, these work by limiting the body's release of histamine, the chemical responsible for relaying the itching sensation.

For the itch, inflammation, and pain that accompany an insect bite or sting, moistened crushed aspirin tablets can be applied to the swollen area. Cold compresses are another natural remedy. Hydrocortisone and hydroacetone creams, lotions, or sprays are probably among the most potent itch-relievers available without prescription.

For those who prefer home remedies or who cannot rush out to a pharmacy at the moment, here are some simple measures to take. Dust cornstarch over wet, weepy rashes to absorb irritating fluids and soothe tender, inflamed skin, or apply a watery paste of oatmeal or baking soda to affected areas. If your body is covered with poison ivy or sunburn, generously lace your tepid bathwater with powdered oatmeal or baking soda. Instead of toweling off, let the solids dry on your skin.

Self-medication for an itch requires a great deal of caution and common sense: The ingredients in salves and lotions designed to soothe or subdue a rash may wind up making the problem worse—particularly if they are formulated in a heavy, greasy base. Besides risking irritation, treating a condition incorrectly will also mask the real problem and prevent an accurate diagnosis, which can lead to costly medical complications later on. For example, scabies is caused by a mite infestation and responds only to a specific medication. Applying any other product will simply prolong the problem.

Boils

When any break in the skin—a sweat or sebaceous gland, hair follicle, or ordinary cut—becomes infected, then rigid, pus-filled (and often painful) lumps are a likely outcome. These also commonly erupt around points of friction caused by clothing such as cuffs and collars, or where chemicals or irritating oils have penetrated skin, and may sometimes be a sign of generally low resistance.

Boils may be few and scattered or many and concentrated, and either small or large; the infection can be short-lived or distressingly persistent. (A carbuncle results when several boils join together so that pus is discharged from several openings of adjacent follicles.) In some cases, pain is severe and hampers movement; the presence of infection can induce fever, malaise, or an elevated white blood-cell count. Most common when the weather is damp, boils can be spread by fingers or clothing and readily transmitted from one person to another.

Boils will usually grow, ripen, and rupture on their own, releasing a fluid containing dead skin, pus, and blood. Most require no more than a simple protective dressing. Warm compresses, applied continuously for at least fifteen minutes, will relieve discomfort and accelerate draining and healing. Your doctor may prescribe an antibiotic ointment to cover the lesions for several days, while penicillin, erythromycin, or tetracycline (an oral antibiotic) is given simultaneously. A germicidal soap may also prove helpful. As with acne, never squeeze a boil; you risk driving the infection deeper into the skin and permanent scarring.

When boils are large, multiple, recurring, or widespread, and especially when they are accompanied by swollen lymph glands and fever, they may point to an underlying systemic disorder. Infected teeth or sinuses and respiratory complications can induce them, so a general checkup is advised in such chronic cases. Since boils have also been associated with diabetes, your doctor may take blood and urine tests, too, as an added precaution.

Cold Sores, Etc.:
Herpes Update

Also called fever blisters and, most recently, "the ulti-
mate parasite," these perplexingly persistent uglies owe
their appearance to two different-but-closely-related viral
infections (herpes simplex) which may invade the skin and
erupt anywhere on the body. Oral herpes or herpes simplex
I affects mostly the lips and mouth, along with the
nose, cheeks and chin, while its dreaded first cousin is the
now raging, near-epidemic· genital herpes (simplex II).
Both disorders announce themselves with itching and often
painful clusters of clear-filled blisters or sores.

In venereal herpes, the lesions may surface in and around
the vagina and on the cervix. In men, the penis and urethra
are targets; in both sexes, the outer thighs and buttocks are
also vulnerable.

Unfortunately, the two viral strains aren't readily distin-
guishable and may easily invade each other's domain.
Researchers have learned belatedly that even the ordinary
cold sore can be transferred to the genitals by fingers or
mouth. In fact, an estimated 15 to 20 percent of all genital
blisters are caused by type I and oral sex is now considered
a major culprit in spreading both varieties. A recent survey
reported in *Time* Magazine shows that one third of women
24 and under who have genital herpes are actually stricken
with the cold sore virus. Likewise, type II sores can also
be transferred to the mouth.

A warning, tingling sensation will usually precede the
blisters by about half a day, and a rather unsightly drying
and crusting stage will occur after the blisters burst and

ooze fluid. The blisters themselves generally appear within two to fifteen days after the initial viral onslaught. In genital herpes, the first bout usually lasts about three weeks and subsequent attacks or recurrences linger roughly five days, sometimes accompanied by fever and painful headaches. Burning urination, watery discharge, swelling of glands or lymph nodes and general malaise are among the other symptoms.

Sometimes the virus makes its entrance without being noticed at all (most likely during early childhood). After breaking the skin barrier, it retreats underground and nests in a nerve root where it may lie dormant indefinitely, or surface at regular intervals. Your body's self-defense system can keep it in check, though emotional and physical stress, illness, injury, infection, fatigue or sun exposure may overcome this built-in immunity and rekindle the virus.

The most contagious period is when the sores and blisters are visible. Avoid close physical and sexual contact during this time and wait until the lesions are completely cleared.

On rare occasions, herpes can journey to the brain, resulting in encephalitis or meningitis, or more commonly, follow another nerve pathway to the eye, triggering an infection which can seriously damage vision if left untreated. In fact, corneal damage due to a herpes virus (ocular herpes) is the leading cause of infectious blindness in the U.S.

Recent Remedies

On the face, the term "cold sore" is technically a misnomer since the problem does not normally coincide with a cold or flu. However, while the sores are not necessarily seasonal, they frequently affect those who are susceptible from November to April, when upper respiratory infections happen to be most prevalent. Occasionally, the blistered skin may become covered with crusts; if these appear stuck on or honey-colored, both staph and strep bacteria may be present and can easily be spread to other parts of the body or to anyone else.

To speed drying and inhibit spreading, cool Burow's soaks, rubbing alcohol, and compresses of cold salt water (1 teaspoon salt to 1 pint water), or all three can help, along with over-the-counter drying preparations. A recently developed product called Resolve, which contains a highly effective anesthetic, is reportedly beneficial and soothing for cold sores during the initial tingling stage even before they erupt. In fact, the odorless, gel-type formula is supposed to work best if applied during this pre-blister period. Never use any hydrocortisone (steroid) cream or ointment after the blisters have appeared, since it may only spread the virus or secondary infection.

Herpaway, another new medicated ointment recently approved by the Food and Drug Administration, is a topically applied solution of tannic, boric, and salicylic acids in an alcohol base. It reportedly yields more than temporary relief, eliminating symptoms and restoring tissue to normal in most cases. Healing time is reduced and discomfort is relieved in four to twelve hours. One of the most recent alternatives, also available now, is 1-Lysine, an over-the-counter tablet that may curb the frequency and severity of herpes viral attacks.

The above medications only help relieve symptoms; they are not antiviral, so you could still be contagious while using such products. A new topical drug called Zovirax (acyclovir) has recently been approved by the Food and Drug Administration as a remedy for cold sores and genital herpes. By singling out infected cells while leaving normal skin intact, acyclovir can reduce pain and discomfort, reportedly prevent new eruptions, speed healing, and limit the time the virus is contagious.

Zovirax is appropriate only for people whose immune

systems have been impaired as a result of chemotherapy or certain illnesses, or those with a first-time case of genital herpes. It has not been FDA-approved for routine use in patients with recurrent cold sores. Not yet a miracle drug in its present form, it appears to work by interfering with the virus' capacity to reproduce.

Preliminary testing with an oral form of the drug shows it to be markedly more effective than the topical kind. Scientists believe that an injectible form of acyclovir will probably offer the best solution for acute cases.

Other encouraging news:

• Researchers at the University of Texas Health Sciences Center in San Antonio have reported that a new experimental anti-herpes formula called BIOF-62 is showing promise in the laboratory and may be tested shortly on human subjects.

• A Los Angeles gynecologist claims a 70 percent success rate using a carbon dioxide laser (which vaporizes herpes lesions) to prevent or delay recurrences.

• Scientists at the Scheie Eye Institute and the University of Pennsylvania in Philadelphia have been testing the therapeutic benefit of a substance called 2-deoxy-D-glucose on women. This topical ointment applied vaginally is believed to halt the spread of herpes simplex viruses by impairing their ability to multiply. So far, tests on subjects with both primary and recurring genital herpes have yielded excellent results.

• Experiments are also being conducted to test the effectiveness of BHT (a food preservative) against genital herpes.

To help you cope and relieve the symptoms, the following guidelines are also recommended:

• Avoid touching sores and blisters to keep from infecting other parts of the body.

• Keep areas clean and dry. Warm baths or wet soaks may soften the affected skin and soothe the irritation, as can cornstarch or talcum powder after thorough drying.

• Wear cotton underwear instead of synthetic fibers which result in excess perspiration.

• Don't wear tight pants since this can aggravate irritation and pain.

• The American Social Health Association has started an information/support service for sufferers. For more details send a self-addressed stamped envelope to HELP, Box 100, Palo Alto, CA 94302.

The organization prints a regular newsletter, conducts group meetings for herpes sufferers, and is involved in disseminating information and keeping its members up-to-date on research and treatment.

Caution for women: There is a strongly suspected, if not yet conclusively proven, link between genital herpes and cervical cancer. For those with either viral strain, once-a-year Pap smears are advised. Even more important, a child born to a woman with an active genital infection has a very great risk of contracting the disease—with most likely dangerous and life-threatening results. To avoid this risk, pregnant women with a history of recurrent genital herpes, those with an active disease during pregnancy, and/or whose sexual partners have proven genital herpes infections should either be delivered by cesarean section or else be carefully monitored through specific laboratory cultures for the presence of the virus before delivery.

Psoriasis

This is certainly not a minor affliction. While never life-threatening, psoriasis can be severely crippling psychologically. Fortunately, some exciting new research appears to be bringing us closer to a cure for this notoriously stubborn disease.

This is how psoriasis happens: For some unknown reason, skin cells start to form and shed at a highly accelerated pace, about six or seven times the usual rate, meaning that it takes about four days instead of twenty-eight for each cell to make its way from the basal (generating) layer of the epidermis to the surface. The result is a piling up of silvery scales over thick, coarse, red patches of skin, either small and discrete or large and widespread. When the scales are removed through rubbing or scratching, tiny pinpoints of bleeding will appear.

While psoriasis may vanish on its own and not return for long periods, there is still no way to prevent its recurrence. And any irritation, infection, or emotional stress can give rise to more flaking and roughness if you are already susceptible.

Despite popular myth, psoriasis is not contagious, nor is it necessarily itchy or uncomfortable. Although there is evidence that it tends to run in families, it cannot be passed from one person to another through bodily contact or by using the same towel or toilet facilities.

What is psoriasis like? In its most common form, it causes a patch of skin to become raised, reddish, itchy, and covered by silvery scales that look something like dandruff. Psoriasis most often appears on the knees, elbows, lower back, buttocks, and scalp, but can occur anywhere. In some, the disease spreads until much of the body is affected. Nails, too, may occasionally be involved; they become thickened, yellowed, and loosened from their beds, marred by pitting and ridging.

Among the factors that can either aggravate or precipitate an outbreak of psoriasis are the following.

An injury to the skin, such as a burn (including severe sunburn), cut, or abrasion may lead to more scaling in one to three weeks.

A change of seasons may cause a variation in intensity. The usual rule is that psoriasis improves in summer and worsens in winter, but there are exceptions.

Psoriasis may intensify during periods of physical or emotional stress.

Bacterial or viral infections, especially those of the upper respiratory tract, along with certain medications, can also aggravate psoriasis.

Psoriasis observes no clear-cut rules or predictable patterns. Thus, very mild cases can suddenly take a turn for the worse, and severe cases can heal spontaneously.

Treatment

Over-the-counter creams, bath products, and shampoos containing coal tars can help reduce dryness and remove the scales. While these preparations are usually straining and medicinal-smelling, new products such as the gel-based Estar or Psorigel are more cosmetically appealing. Chemicals such as salicylic acid can also peel away scales and allow for better absorption of other medications. These are especially well absorbed if the skin is moistened first, then covered securely with clear plastic after being treated.

Sunlight is probably one of the most dramatic remedies of all. Many psoriasis sufferers report striking improvement during summer months, especially after long periods of sunbathing. (Constant sun exposure may well explain why the face is generally least affected by psoriasis.) For years dermatologists and hospital clinics have treated hard-to-cure patients with light boxes, special booths lined with mylar (a silver reflective surface) and cylindrical bulbs emitting short-wave ultraviolet radiation (also called ultraviolet B rays or UVBs). Recently a group of medical centers has been studying the effects of long-wave radiant energy (called ultraviolet A rays or UVAs) on people who have also been treated with a safe, well-tested drug compound known as a psoralen. This chemical enhances the absorption of the UVAs and combines with them to slow down the growth and turnover rate of explosively peeling skin cells by affecting their DNA makeup. (The combination therapy is called PUVA, which stands for psoralen plus UVA.)

Two hours after taking a psoralen pill, allowing time for its absorption into the bloodstream and transportation to the skin, the patient is exposed to the light box for a carefully prescribed period (to prevent burning and skin damage). This ritual is repeated two or three times a week until all the psoriasis clears, usually after about eight to twelve weeks. PUVA, the most promising treatment so far, has recently been approved for widespread use by the

FDA. However, it is not without some risk, especially for people with very fair skin or a previous history of X ray treatment or skin cancer, who may be more susceptible than usual to sunlight's damaging effects.

New evidence reveals that psoriasis clears more quickly and with smaller doses of ultraviolet light when a strong topical corticosteroid chemical is added to the PUVA treatment. According to this study, combination therapy may save the patient time, money, and unnecessary exposure to radiant energy. While clearing occurs with both methods, the PUVA plus topical treatment is much faster.

When UVB (ultraviolet burning radiation) is combined with PUVA, the rate of healing is also dramatically increased. This equally new dual therapy reduces total ultraviolet exposure by half, which can lessen the possible side effects of such treatment, namely skin cancer.

There has been yet another breakthrough. The Third International Psoriasis Symposium, held at Stanford University, reported on a new synthetic (and still experimental) form of vitamin A called an aromatic retinoid, which has been remarkably effective against severe cases of psoriasis. It, too, can accelerate healing when used in combination with PUVA. The new hope is that one or two convenient, daily, potent yet risk-free retinoid pills—described as one of the most exciting drugs in the history of dermatology— may soon replace the clumsy creams and lotions that are still an inescapable ritual for too many psoriasis victims.

A class of drugs called antimetabolites slow the growth rate of cells by interfering with their metabolism. The most common example among these agents is methotrexate; while beneficial in certain severe cases, it is still under careful scrutiny, because it can inhibit the growth of normal cells, too. Some natural substances apparently slow the cell-growth rate as well. One such compound is CAMP 9 (short for cyclic adenosine monophosphate). Unfortunately it does not penetrate cells effectively enough, though experiments are now under way to increase its potency and that of similar drugs.

Another possible treatment for psoriasis, currently the subject of study at Stanford University, involves heating by ultrasound. As with PUVA, the use of ultrasound heating (also called controlled hyperthermia) was prompted by the simple observation that the disease often improves in summer, whether or not the patient has been exposed to sunlight—meaning the heat must be an important healing factor. In preliminary tests so far, thirteen out of twenty-one people were completely cleared of psoriasis, and the effects lasted up to two or three months without further treatment. Six cases showed partial improvement, and only two remained unaffected. While it is too early to compare hyperthermia with other methods, it is believed this method works best when the scaly patches are small and confined.

Topical corticosteroid creams or coal tar pastes sealed tightly by a synthetic plastic wrapping or a polyethylene film have been among the traditional therapies for psoriasis. But the covering itself often results in excessive sweating and discomfort. One novel alternative is a disposable yet durable paper jumpsuit, which is light and allows the patient's topically treated skin to breathe, a welcome advantage during the summer. No staining occurs through the paper as it does with ordinary cloth pajamas, which can no longer be used or washed when smeared with coal tar or anthralin paste.

Note: If you are battling a lingering case, check out the special psoriasis day-care centers in your city or region, where your condition can be bombarded with a multiple offensive: topical lotions, shampoos, special baths, and possibly PUVA—entailing far less expense than any local hospital.

Note: Adverse effects of PUVA therapy include nausea, vomiting, dizziness, pruritis (itching), headache, uneven or excessive tanning, drying, freckling and peeling, and severe swelling. Among the possible results of long-term treatment are accelerated aging of the skin, skin cancers, undesirable changes in the immune system, and cataracts (preventable by wearing protective goggles upon taking psoralen and wearing sunglasses up to eight hours after treatment).

One follow up study of more than 1,300 patients treated with PUVA showed the incidence of skin cancer to be twice that expected of the general population. After four years the basal cell cancer rate was 1.8 times higher than normal, while that for squamous cell cancer was nine times the usual rate. In both diseases, tumors also appeared in areas of the skin not previously exposed to sunlight.

Pigmentation Problems

Melasma

Melasma (also called chloasma, gravidarum, or the mask of pregnancy) is the term for mottled, liver-spotted skin, especially on the face, forehead, and temples. These flat, smooth, brownish, and entirely harmless blemishes, larger than freckles and up to several inches in diameter, can be triggered by repeated sun exposure, oral contraceptives, or pregnancy. While they often disappear spontaneously, complete clearing may take up to a year. If the condition is caused by pregnancy, it usually clears within a few months of delivery. However, melasma resulting from the Pill has been known to last up to five years after a woman has stopped using oral contraceptives, because current treatment is still far from satisfactory.

Use sunscreens to prevent them and bleaching creams (preferably the prescription kind) containing hydroquinone to help fade them away. Sunscreens should always be used during bleaching treatment. If you insist on having them removed, freezing with liquid nitrogen or dry ice can lighten pigment after only one or two sessions. Your dermatologist may also resort to the reliable electric needle or to a mild acid followed by a specially prepared bleaching formula.

Pitryasis Rosea: Mysterious, Not Serious

You can't catch it, it rarely ever strikes twice, it seldom itches, and almost always vanishes on its own without treatment: This happily harmless, short-lived nuisance, called *pityriasis rosea* (often mistaken for ringworm) generally starts out as a single large pinkish patch called the "mother" or "herald." Smaller round or oval offspring lesions emerge within about two weeks and spread over chest and back. Though it usually disappears without a trace after six or eight weeks, the rash may darken skin temporarily, especially in brunettes.

If itching does occur, tepid baths and bath oils or an oral antihistamine can provide relief. (Avoid all but the mildest soaps to reduce irritation.)

Vitiligo

An abrupt, unexplained loss of pigment, caused by the sudden departure of pigment-producing cells, describes this curious condition. The bleached-out areas appear as distinctly outlined patches of all sizes and shapes, and may become widespread, originating from almost anywhere: the scalp, sites of injury, or segments of skin that are supplied by a nerve. Patches of hair, too, may become stripped of color. Excessive sunburn is a possible catalyst, while infection, illness, and emotional difficulty can all intensify an existing problem. While vitiligo strikes mostly people in otherwise good general health, the disorder occurs with higher than average frequency in those with one of the following conditions: hyperthyroidism or increased thyroid gland function, Addison's disease (which affects the adrenal glands), alopecia areata (patchy, usually temporary hair loss), and pernicious anemia (vitamin B_{12} deficiency).

While no one has yet solved the riddle, two theories about the origins of vitiligo are currently popular. One points to a possible abnormality in the nerve endings near pigment cells within the skin and hair follicles. According to this explanation, the natural graying of hair, which results from a loss of ability to form melanin, is part of a similar (vitiliginous) process. Thus, the type of phenomenon that halts pigment formation in the hair may also be responsible for blocking the production of melanin in the skin.

The other theory suggests that vitiligo is an autoimmune condition in which the sufferer becomes allergic to his or her own pigment or parts of pigment cells, thus losing the capacity to manufacture melanin.

In the fair-skinned, the onset of vitiligo is generally more conspicuous during the summer, when the contrast between bleached-out and sunburned areas is especially striking; in the dark-skinned, of course, the condition is highly visible all year round. The loss of pigment is not necessarily consistent or uniform, even within a single patch of vitiligo. Thus, varying shades can mark a given affected area.

Often the disease runs a cyclical course—a rapid loss of pigment followed by periods of prolonged stability—an alternating pattern that may go on for years. Only rarely does a person with vitiligo regain color spontaneously.

Some people are good candidates for repigmentation therapy (restoration of color). In general, children and young adults respond best, especially if they have had the condition less than five years. Motivation and willingness to persevere in an often time-consuming treatment is also necessary for success. No one with sensitivity or allergy to sunlight should be a candidate.

Treatment

Under a doctor's supervision, a psoralen pill (methoxy or trimethyl psoralen) is administered orally about one or two hours before the patient goes out in the sun (preferably when ultraviolet rays are most concentrated, between 11 A.M. and 1 P.M., May through September, in the northern part of the United States). PUVA is also being used to treat vitiligo. After the first exposure to ultraviolet light, the vitiligo will actually look worse, because the discolored areas will appear even more bleached by contrast with the newly tanned skin. However, repigmentation will gradually take place in the patches, either as pigment spreads from adjoining areas, or in the form of central spots of color that gradually enlarge with continued exposure.

Some physicians apply topical solutions of psoralens directly to the light patches before exposing patients to sunlight. When the spots are small and scattered, this approach works well. The chief drawback is that the pigment-stimulating medication makes the skin more photosensitive, meaning that it is at higher risk of severe burns and blisters if overexposed, a process that is hard to control.

Until skin color returns, dark-shaded cream foundations and makeups, such as Covermark, will camouflage well. For men who object to makeup, two types of stains may be just as effective cosmetically. One called dihydroxyacetone is a colorless solution that combines with proteins in the outer layers of skin to impart a tan surface color. It is available in concentrations of up to five percent in several products. Another type of product consists of an aniline dye or walnut juice, sometimes in combination with dihydroxyacetone. While it is difficult to stain the skin evenly and match normal skin precisely, many patients are pleased with the results, even while they are undergoing psoralen treatment. (The two don't clash.)

Sometimes when pigment loss is extensive—over fifty percent of the body—restoring color may be all but impossible. In this case, some doctors try to depigment the rest of the body for consistency. This is accomplished with the application to the skin of a special chemical agent, such as hydroquinone, once or twice daily during the winter months. During summer, skin should be protected constantly with a total sunblock cream. Obviously, the disadvantage of this method is that it leaves patients far less tolerant of exposure to the sun.

Keratoses

Seborrheic keratoses
These are simply benign, pigmented overgrowths of the outer layers of skin. Waxlike, loosely raised, and either rounded or irregular, they erupt alone or in clusters in all different colors, usually brownish, and seem stuck or pasted on the skin. They take root most commonly on the trunk, face, and scalp, and their size and number may increase gradually with age. Since these are neither potentially cancerous nor contagious, they are best left alone unless they become irritated or infected.

Not caused by sunlight, seborrheic keratoses appear on both covered and uncovered parts of the body. Generally, the growths begin as slightly raised light-brown spots. Eventually these thicken and assume a rough, wartlike texture. They also darken slowly and may turn black, a completely harmless change. Why these blemishes appear is unknown. Sometimes they break out during pregnancy or after estrogen therapy or on skin that has recently recovered from an inflammatory disorder. Their occurrence in members of the same family suggests an inherited condition. Since they are no cause for concern, the only reason for having them removed (quickly and painlessly curetted, electrically singed, or frozen away in the doctor's office) is if they are unattractive, conspicuous, itchy, or continually rubbing against clothes or jewelry.

Note: The *sudden* appearance of seborrheic keratoses may herald an underlying malignancy, especially adenocarcinoma (Leser-Trelat disease).

Solar or actinic keratoses

These have a markedly grainy or sandy surface and are firmly anchored to the skin. The sun-exposed portions of the body—face, hands, forearms, and V of the neck—are the most favored targets for these blemishes, which are induced by overexposure to solar radiation. The pale-skinned, fair-haired, and light-eyed are especially susceptible.

If left untreated, these sun spots, unlike the seborrheic variety, may turn malignant. For this reason, any raised, reddish, scaly, sandy-textured lesions should be evaluated by a dermatologist. Since most actinic keratoses are superficial, treatment is relatively simple and nonscarring. Removal involves spraying or daubing with liquid nitrogen to freeze and destroy affected cells and encourage mild peeling (cryosurgery); sparking with a weak electric current through a needle and/or surgical scraping (curettage) or excision; or chemical treatment with an agent such as topical 5-fluorouracil (5 FU), which is selectively absorbed by pre-malignant areas and especially appropriate if you have a cluster or large concentration of lesions on the face, upper extremities, V of the chest, back of the neck, and scalp. The topical chemical is rubbed on as a cream or lotion twice a day over a two to three week period.

Sometimes psoriasis or seborrheic dermatitis may be difficult to distinguish from superficial actinic keratoses. In this case your doctor may choose to treat the skin with a topical corticosteroid cream for several weeks and then reevaluate the condition. Any dermatitis usually responds to this regimen, while keratoses undergo very little change.

Keep in mind that once sun damage has progressed to the point where these blemishes develop, new ones may appear after treatment, even without further sun exposure. (For the complete story on the skin damage wrought by sun, see Chapter 1.)

Prevention is by far the best policy. If you are fair-complexioned, stay out of the sun as often as possible, especially between 10 A.M. and 2 P.M. in a temperate zone; wear a hat in summer, carry a sunscreen—and use it faithfully.

Seborrheic Dermatitis

In its mildest form—popularly known as dandruff—this most common of complaints is marked by persistent though patchy peeling and flaking of the scalp. A severe case can also lead to redness, scaling, and possible bacterial infection of the eyebrows, eyelids, sides of the nose, chest, and upper back, even the navel and around the groin. Sometimes the disorder so closely resembles psoriasis (and vice versa) that the ambiguous term "seborrhiasis" has been coined to describe it.

While the exact cause of seborrheic dermatitis is unknown, dermatologists suspect a hormone imbalance, microorganisms, or an oil gland disorder, with heredity as a more than likely predisposer (flakiness probably runs in families!). Diabetes, heavy drinking, obesity, and respiratory infections can all aggravate the condition, as can spells of nervous tension and fatigue. Often seborrheic dermatitis accompanies a case of severe acne or rosacea.

Regular shampooing with nonprescription medicated products (which typically contain selenium sulfide, tar, sulfur, zinc pyrithione, or some antibacterial agent) can lead to marked improvement, along with salicylic acid, resorcinol, or cortisone in the form of a lotion, cream, or spray. Switching or rotating shampoos routinely is a good strategy since your scalp may become immune to a given formula. For best results, massage the product well into the scalp, rinse, then repeat. Let shampoo soak in for five minutes before rinsing off again thoroughly to remove all traces of soapy film. Soaps and other residues of medicated products can act as a glue that clumps small flakes together to form larger, more visible ones.

This largely seasonal disorder is active or dormant, depending on the time of year. During the winter and early spring, for example, you may need to shampoo every day, while only a once- or twice-weekly cleansing might well be sufficient later on. Summer often brings about a natural remission before the condition flares up again in the fall. When outbreaks are severe, your doctor may prescribe an oral medication temporarily.

Blonds are less likely to have scaling scalps than either brunettes or redheads; people of Irish descent are especially susceptible. Even newborn babies aren't immune. A temporary syndrome known as cradle cap, possibly triggered by circulating maternal hormones, can be bothersome during the first few months. But after this clears, children up to the age of puberty are almost never affected. (This lends some credibility to the hormone/oil gland theories.)

As for dandruff, it is not a dry-scalp condition even though the individual flakes appear to be parched. In most cases, dandruff scales are actually oily, so applying greases and oils to the scalp only makes matters worse, even while it momentarily camouflages the problem. Some dermatologists believe that dandruff is neither a disease nor simply a mild version of seborrheic dermatitis, but rather a normal physiological, noninflammatory phenomenon, much like the growth of hair and nails. But however it is described, its visibility often makes it distressing and, to many, socially unacceptable.

Shingles

Shingles or herpes zoster is caused by the same virus that gives rise to chicken pox, marked by a blistery, itching outbreak. After you're exposed to chicken pox, the virus remains dormant in the body within the nerve cells lining the spinal cord. Then later in life the virus may be reactivated or travel along the sensory nerves to the skin and cause extremely painful blisters or eruptions.

The tiny lesions come in clusters surrounded by tender, irritated skin and are usually confined to one side of the body. When the blisters finally break, a scab or crust forms over the dried-out fluids. Pain may precede their appearance, and it may persist long after the eruptions have cleared (a condition called post-herpetic neuralgia). Fatigue, fever, and headache are also possible complications.

For days, even weeks, before the first visible signs appear, an aching or burning feeling may emanate from the area nourished by the affected nerve. This region— beginning at the spine and extending down one side of the body or traveling along a limb—is known as a dermatome. The pain and itching, often intense, usually trace the path of the underlying nerves.

Fifteen-minute soaks with compresses dipped in salted tepid water (a teaspoon of salt per pint of water) help dry blisters and stave off infection. They should be applied every four to six hours. Antibiotics, antihistamines, and analgesics can be used for infection, itching, and pain. Calamine lotion will help relieve itching and soothe the affected tissues, as will creams or injections containing steroids (used for a strictly limited period of time). When shingles occurs on the side of the nose, an ophthalmologist should be consulted promptly to make sure the eye has not been affected. If shingles has infected the eye area, special eye drops and other treatment may be necessary.

While theoretically anyone who has had chicken pox can contract the disease, shingles often strikes when a person's defenses are at their lowest, following a major illness or surgery or extreme emotional stress.

Scabies

This is a contagious and increasingly common condition, the cause of which is both specific and very much alive: a family of mites lodging under the skin that lays its eggs and multiplies. The body reacts to these unwanted intruders by breaking out in groups of red, itching bumps, commonly found between the fingers or circling the wrist, around the nipples, armpits, waist, elbows, or knees, the genital area, buttocks, back, or outer borders of the feet. People who travel or camp out a great deal are probably more susceptible than usual.

The disease has plagued man for thousands of years; ancient Greeks and Romans described the annoying itch in their records. Historically, epidemics of the disease have been particularly common during crowded wartime conditions. By the 1950s, scabies here and abroad declined rapidly to the point at which one medical dictionary defined it as a "now extinct" organism. Recently, however, for reasons not yet clear, scabies has been making a vigorous comeback in the United States.

Unlike many other skin disorders, scabies does not discriminate on the basis of age, race, sex, or place of residence. Virtually anyone can fall victim: business executive, soldier, physician, housewife, college student, teenager, or infant. How do you get the disease? Very easily, since it is highly catching. Scabies often spreads among family members, roommates, and sexual partners quite rapidly due to their close contact. Exchanging clothing or sharing a bed or towels is also a means of spreading the condition.

How does scabies happen? The male and female mite mate on the surface of the skin. Then the female burrows under the outermost layer, leaving a trail of eggs behind her. In a few days the eggs hatch and the larvae travel to the surface. Here they grow into mites, which start the mating and egg-laying cycle all over again once they reach maturity. While the mites themselves are extremely difficult to see without a magnifying glass, the linear, zigzag burrows are often quite visible to the naked eye, typically appearing as grayish-white threads. If your doctor suspects scabies, he will look for these trails wherever you complain of an itch or swelling. To confirm his diagnosis, he may want to scrape a few tiny specks of skin from the itchy area (a quick, painless procedure), place the specimen on a slide, and examine it under a microscope.

The first time you catch the disease it takes about four weeks from the moment of infestation for the symptoms to emerge. Sometimes the mites can be spread before you feel the slightest discomfort, which is why scabies can be spread before anyone is yet aware of the problem. Once symptoms announce themselves, you will probably feel the most intense itching during the night, when the mites are believed to be most active. Some people with scabies feel dirty and take frequent scalding showers; however, this only dries out the skin and intensifies the itching.

See your doctor immediately if you believe you or someone in your family has scabies. If you have the disease, he will probably prescribe a cream or lotion containing lindane, sold under such trade names as Kwell and Scabene, which kills the mites when applied to the skin. Follow usage instructions carefully. Bathe before applying the medication and then cover your body with a thin coating from the neck down, smearing affected areas more heavily. Do not apply the lindane to your face or scalp and be very careful to avoid contact with your eyes. Wash off thoroughly twelve hours later. Usually one application will rout the pests within twenty-four hours. Your doctor may instruct you to reapply the medication in one week. However, even after successful treatment, the itching may continue for another week or two. Do not reapply medication unless your doctor explicitly instructs you to do so. Your doctor may also prescribe an antihistamine to help relieve itching. Another effective medication for scabies called crotamiton (Eurax) will help curb itching on contact with skin and also kill the scabies mites.

Unfortunately, you cannot become immune to scabies. Since scabies is easily transmitted, make sure family members and sex partners are treated all at the same time so as to avoid passing the disease back and forth.

Dilated Blood Vessels

These spidery red lines, sometimes incorrectly referred to as broken capillaries, are entirely harmless but all too often visible beneath thin, dry facial skin, especially near the eyes, cheeks, and sides of nostrils. Treatment is via electric needle (electrodesiccation), which blanches vessels instantly and coagulates the blood. The capillary walls then disintegrate and disappear. Usually a fine crust or scab will form over the treated area, followed by temporary discoloration. Since there is a two in ten chance that the capillary will return, the procedure may have to be repeated.

Excessive sun exposure, vitamin C deficiency, hot showers, extremes of temperature, too much alcohol, pregnancy, high blood pressure, facial massage, and trauma are among the causes. To help prevent this condition, wear a sunscreen regularly, do not use harsh cosmetics, eat plenty of fresh fruits and vegetables, and take daily supplements of vitamin C.

In stubborn cases, dilated vessels can also be swiftly and bloodlessly beamed away with a selective, color-coded argon laser. An office procedure currently in limited use, this approach sends forth a blue-green light that causes a reaction only in red-colored areas. This makes it perfect for singling out distended capillaries and prominent wine-stained or strawberry birthmarks.

Stretch Marks

When skin is stretched for long periods, as a result of pregnancy or obesity, for example, or repeated, rapid fluctuations in weight, the elastic fibers that give the deeper layers resiliency and strength lose their natural spring. (Think of a rubber band that has been played with too often and irreversibly distended out of shape.) What shows up on the surface are striae or the notorious stretch marks:

linear, grooved, or crescent-shaped depressions, colored red or dusky bluish, that gradually fade with time.

They appear in areas of the body where skin is subject to repeated pulling or expansion—buttocks, abdomen, thighs, hips, breasts. About twenty percent of adolescent girls and ten percent of normal-weight men show areas of stretch-marked skin, particularly on the lumbar region of the back. Wrestlers and weight lifters may have them, too, across the shoulders and on the back. Along with mechanical stress, hormones are believed to play a leading role, the reason stretch marks plague so many more women than men.

Aside from weight gain and childbearing, exposure to topical or systemic corticosteroid drugs could permanently thin the outer and inner layers, resulting in atrophy and a decrease in both collagen and elastin, the proteins that normally buttress the skin. It is best to consult a dermatologist for stretch marks, since diagnosis can pose a problem; these uglies have been mistaken for disorders, and vice versa.

Many women are so upset by stretch marks that they fall easy prey to false promises and bogus claims: *No* topical cream or medication can eliminate them, nor has any internal antidote yet been devised! So far, a good camouflaging makeup, well-matched to your skin tone, is the best solution. Heavy theatrical makeups, coversticks or several coats of cream-based liquid cosmetics are especially effective concealers. Fortunately, stretch marks fade normally, eventually turning a nearly imperceptible white. Of course, plastic surgeons can excise flabby skin and tighten muscles, and possibly dermabrade the affected area as well, but these are drastic approaches that may trade in a simple cosmetic problem for permanent, unsightly scars.

Besides good cosmetics, prevention is by far the best policy. This means not gaining too many extra pounds during pregnancy, or any other time and avoiding prolonged straining or pressure on parts of the body, or long-term use of corticosteroids. In the future, dermatologists may choose to plump out the most stubborn, deep-seated stretch marks with collagen implants, which are now showing such promise in the treatment of shallow acne scars and fine wrinkles (see Chapters 6 and 8).

Unwanted Hair

In our society, facial and bodily hair on a woman is considered both unattractive and unfeminine. Sometimes the problem of *excessive* hair growth can be traced to malfunctioning adrenal glands. To simplify: The adrenal glands produce hormones, one of which is androgen. Though known as the male hormone, androgen is manufactured in women's bodies, too. It plays an important role in bone development, regulates the secretion of sebum from the skin's oil glands, and is crucial in determining sexual characteristics, including the amount and consistency of facial hair. When there are high levels of androgen in a woman's body, the result may be an overgrowth—or hirsutism, as it is more properly called.

During puberty, when glands are working overtime, a young girl's body may become "confused" and produce excessive androgen. Girls with this problem characteristically have erratic menstrual periods, underdeveloped breasts, and too much facial hair.

A dermatologist can determine whether adrenal malfunction is the underlying cause. When the problem is successfully treated, the unwanted hair often falls out on its own, and regrowth is minimal.

In fact, glandular problems are rather rare. Most women afflicted with unwanted hair simply have inherited the genes for it. Some ethnic groups, especially those of Mediterranean ancestry, tend to be hairier than others. However, many brunettes are distressed by what they think is excessive hair, when actually they have no more than usual. Their hair is dark and therefore more noticeable.

Hair can be removed by shaving, waxing, rubbing with pumice, chemical depilatories, plucking, and electrolysis or camouflaged by bleaching.

Shaving is a cheap, simple, rapid, and temporary method of hair removal, which does not destroy the hair below the surface. For best results, you have to do it regularly and often—at least once or twice a week. (There is absolutely no truth to the notion that frequent shaving causes hair to grow back thicker or more rapidly.) If your skin is sensitive, first smooth on some olive oil or moisturizing cream. Then use a good lathery soap or shaving cream to help keep you from getting nicked. Reapply moisturizer afterward to prevent dryness.

Waxing, an efficient way of removing hair from large areas, is a longer-lasting alternative. In this procedure, melted wax is spread on the skin and allowed to dry and harden. Then it is stripped off. Hair caught in the hardened wax is removed along with it. Because waxing pulls hair out from the roots, new growth is slow to appear (it may take as long as six weeks).

This method works well for legs, for hair on your upper lip and chin, between your brows, under your arms, or at the bikini line. And it is not difficult to do yourself. Having it done at a salon is a lot easier, however, and often more comfortable; when an expert does it, there is no more sting than you feel when you rip a Band-Aid off very quickly.

If you prefer to do it at home, apply warm wax in the direction in which the hair is growing. Cover with a strip of muslin, then pull off quickly in the other direction, going against the grain of the hair.

The more you wax an area, the less the hair is apt to grow back, since waxing tends to damage the hair follicle.

Chemical depilatories are creams, lotions, sprays, and foams that soften hair to the point at which it can be wiped off the skin. Depilatories work well on upper lip, legs, and underarms; new hair growth appears within a week or so and often feels less coarse. Keep in mind that depilatories can irritate the skin. Be sure to do a patch test (described on p. 164) to determine whether your skin can tolerate it before applying the depilatory all over.

Rubbing and plucking have some disadvantages. Although rubbing with a pumice is an effective method, it may be too rough for the delicate skin on your face. Tweezing or plucking pulls the hair out, but is impractical for large areas. It is painful, can cause inflammation, and may damage the hair, resulting in coarser growth.

Electrolysis is the only permanent method of hair removal. The procedure involves the use of a very fine needle, which is inserted in a hair follicle. Electric current passing through the needle to the root of the hair destroys the papilla. As a result, no new hair grows from the follicle.

Electrolysis can be expensive. Several half-hour or hour-long treatments may be required, depending on how much hair is to be cleared. There is also some pain, though many people who have undergone electrolysis say it is no more uncomfortable than waxing or tweezing. You should avoid using makeup for a couple of hours or more if you have had the procedure done on your face. Just use a mild calamine lotion to soothe and protect the skin.

New on the scene is the IB probe, a needle with silicon insulation along its shaft and an uninsulated bulbous tip. The bulbous tip assures that the needle enters the skin only at a follicle opening; the insulation insures that current is discharged only on contact with the papilla. Thus, the IB probe is said to be more efficient and less painful than a regular needle. The probe is also flexible, which makes it more effective in treating follicles distorted by waxing or tweezing.

People who wear a cardiac pacemaker are not good

candidates for electrolysis; diabetics should take great care, since they are more susceptible to infection. Neither is the procedure recommended for girls under sixteen or for blacks because of hyper pigmentation. For others, though, it may be the best solution to the unwanted hair problem.

It is important that the electrologist be competent, experienced, and a graduate of an accredited school, or else infection and scarring can possibly result. Ask your family doctor, endocrinologist, or dermatologist to recommend a good one. (You can verify credentials by writing to the education department of the state where the electrologist's school is located.)

Bleaching can be an excellent solution for areas such as the upper lip and the arms where the hair is short and fine or dark but not profuse. You can buy bleaching products (containing peroxide and ammonia plus a little mild soap) and do the job at home or you can have it done at a salon. Be sure to do a patch test inside the elbow before applying the product all over. Before and after bleaching, use a moisturizing lotion to soften the skin.

Hair Loss

At first, the thirty-eight-year-old mother of two who held down a demanding job as an insurance claims adjuster was only mildly concerned about her thinning hair. She had more important matters to worry about than the hundreds of strands that came out in her comb each morning. But when she discovered a progressively enlarging area of baldness on the top of her head, Mary had to face facts. She was going bald.

The problem worsened. "There was a time," she recalls with wry humor, "when I felt like Joe Garagiola in a dress." That was a couple of years ago. Today Mary's hair is thicker, and she is free of bald spots, thanks to the surgical procedure that has helped so many balding men to look and feel better about themselves.

More and more women each year are considering hair transplants (described below). Some, like Mary, have symptoms of what is called male pattern balding (the Joe Garagiola look). Much more common in both sexes is overall thinning of the hair. Both types of hair loss may fall into the category of androgenic baldness, which seems to be on the rise in women.

The hairs on your head are constantly being shed and replaced at the rate of fifty to a hundred a day, a normal process as new growth pushes its way to the surface. Hair also naturally thins with age as a result of hormone changes, although this is usually imperceptible and not a cosmetic concern.

Abnormal hair loss can be an isolated, temporary episode, a recurring problem, or a chronic, lingering disorder. Some women inherit strong genes for baldness from one or both parents. You might say they are programmed for baldness, and as years go by they may begin to lose some or a great deal of hair, especially from the sides and top of the scalp. Others may or may not have the troublesome baldness genes but do not lose their hair unless or until something triggers an increase in male hormones in their bodies.

That "something" could be emotional stress, which can raise the level of male hormones in women. In fact, the tense times we live in could well be responsible for the rise in female androgenic baldness. Other culprits can be found among the one hundred and forty-odd pharmaceuticals—including wheat germ oil and some birth control pills—that are also male hormone stimulants. (Oddly, these same androgenic drugs are also often a factor in both acne and hirsutism; the one brings too much oil and the other too much hair to the face and body, where neither is welcome.) While mostly associated with midlife, the hair-thinning syndrome can begin well before, sometimes even in the late twenties and early thirties.

Alopecia areata is a nonscarring, usually temporary hair loss marked by round or oval patches of baldness. Most cases involve only a few such spots, and hair stops being shed after a few weeks. Alopecia's sudden onset may follow a trauma or shock to the body—pregnancy, crash dieting, emotional stress, high fever, major illnesses such as thyroid disease, diabetes, and anemia, certain systemic drugs such as cholesterol-reducers, agents used in chemotherapy, steroids, and amphetamines.

Paradoxically, paying too much attention to your hair may also increase your chances of losing it. Coloring, straightening, drying, frequent shampooing, brushing or conditioning, using tight curlers or clasps, or repeated pulling and twisting. Cold wave solutions without a built-in neutralizer can have a depilatory (hair-removing) effect if they are left on too long. Very severe dandruff or seborrheic dermatitis may occasionally strip away hairs, as may psoriasis, boils, shingles, and other skin disorders.

Although alopecia is usually short-lived, stubborn cases may respond readily to low-dose cortisone injections directly into the scalp. Regrowth, light and fine-textured at first, begins within several weeks and remains confined to the injected area. Sometimes topical applications of steroids under airtight plastic wrappings are an equally effective way to "fertilize" the scalp again. Doctors have reported promising results with estrogen or progesterone lotions, progesterone drops, progesterone injections, and thyroid hormones given orally. Psychotherapy is an attempted "cure" for hair loss induced by anxiety and stress.

To minimize hair loss anytime, always use a gentle hand. Avoid zealous combing, especially when hair is wet, since this pulls strands out by their roots or along their shafts, or ruptures them from the scalp. Limit brushing, too, and always use natural bristles instead of nylon ones.

When either combing or brushing, hold the hair part way between its tip and your scalp to reduce tension and prevent breakage. Regular mild shampooing can help preserve hair and even stimulate growth. Perhaps one reason is that it flushes away squalene, an ingredient found in scalp oil that actually removes hair (nature's own depilatory!).

Pattern Baldness: New Solutions

New, highly experimental research points to a possible drug solution in the future for the more severe, so far incurable pattern baldness. Scientists have discovered that most of the testosterone (male hormone) present in both men and women is bound up by a natural liver protein called TGB. The remainder circulates freely and finds its way to special cells in the hair follicles. There an enzyme converts the liberated testosterone into a more potent, troublesome form called didydrotestosterone. This drives some follicles to sprout new hairs while shutting down others completely. The result is often too little hair on the head and too much on the face.

An excess of the freewheeling testosterone in the bloodstream may simply result from a deficiency of the binding protein. Researchers have found that oral thyroid supplements apparently spur the liver to manufacture more of the necessary protein. They are also developing new drugs: Some block testosterone's conversion to the more powerful form, while others "confuse" the conversion enzyme or prevent the male hormone from entering those hair follicle cells where it can do the most damage.

However, until such drugs are proven safe and are available for widespread use, hair transplants are probably the best alternative. Hair weaving, hair implantation, and fiber implants are other choices, but all have serious drawbacks. In hair weaving, the patient's own hair is used to anchor a woven-on hairpiece to the scalp. The technique tends to weaken and damage what is left of the wearer's hair. Not only that but also the process needs to be repeated frequently, since the hairpiece will loosen and lift as the patient's locks grow longer.

Hair implantation, in which a hairpiece is sutured to the scalp, can result in lingering soreness and lead to scarring that may destroy some of the patient's healthy hair follicles. Ordinary combing, styling, and shampooing tend to loosen and pull out implanted hair.

Fiber implants, the introduction of synthetic fibers into the scalp, can have such disastrous consequences—infection, scarring, soreness, and facial swelling—that the procedure is now being closely scrutinized by the United States Food and Drug Administration.

In a hair transplant, the patient's own healthy hair follicles are taken from areas of the scalp where hair is thick and relocated in balding areas, where they eventually sprout and grow normally. Transplantation can be an excellent technique when baldness is the result of burns or scars, including scars in the sideburn and temple areas that are the aftermath of face-lift surgery.

In simplified terms, this is how the method works. After a thorough shampooing, hair is clipped from the donor area of the scalp (the section from which hair follicles will be taken). A local anesthetic is administered, then a small tool about four millimeters in diameter—something like a miniature cookie cutter—is used to cut tiny sections or plugs of skin from the donor area. Anywhere from fifty to sixty plugs may be cut at this time. Next an equal number of plugs is cut from the bald area, leaving a series of small indentations or holes. Donor plugs are trimmed and fitted into holes.

Stitches or sutures are rarely necessary to keep the plugs in place. Bleeding is minimal and controlled by pressure. When it has stopped, the head is loosely bandaged and the patient can go home. Next day the patient returns to the office for a progress check. Bandages are removed, and the whole head is rinsed and dried.

The clipped hair stubs in the transplanted plugs do not immediately begin to grow. Instead, they fall out within a few weeks of the operation. Then for a while—nothing. Hair follicles are resting up after the trauma of relocation. This resting phase sometimes lasts for as long as twenty weeks. In the meantime, the patient can go about his or her ordinary business, wear a hat or hairpiece, shampoo and style the rest of the hair as usual, and even go swimming (though it is not a good idea to allow the scalp to become sunburned).

Finally new hair begins to sprout in the transplant area. It will be the same color as hair in the area from which it was taken, but at first may be somewhat coarser in texture. (The coarseness is a plus, since coarse hair appears thicker than baby-fine hair.) The new hair will grow at the same rate as hair on the rest of the head and will eventually blend in with it. When it is long enough, transplanted hair may be styled, cut, colored, permed, and straightened, just like ordinary hair. In fact, it *is* just ordinary hair.

Those fifty to sixty plugs transplanted in the first session may not be enough, however, to make a real difference. A second, third, and even fourth session may be necessary, depending on the size of the balding areas to be filled in and the patient's expectations. Most dermatologists charge on a per plug basis at a rate of $10 to $25 for each. Usually at least four sessions are required, so the procedure can be costly. But to the women who say they feel younger, more attractive, and as one thirty-five-year-old puts it, "just all around psychologically better," the money is well spent.

Only a dermatologist can tell for sure whether someone is a good candidate for a hair transplant. The doctor's first job is to determine the type and cause of the patient's hair loss. Not until then can any particular treatment be suggested. For example, with certain types of alopecia areata, the entire scalp is potentially at risk for the disease, so there are no clear-cut donor sites. However, if the disease persists after treatment and is no longer progressive (showing signs of getting worse), a hair transplant attempt may be worthwhile.

The transplant procedure, although not painful, may be

upsetting to the squeamish. Hypnosis can serve as a kind of natural tranquilizer for patients with delicate stomachs; results are usually excellent.

Hair and skin type need to be considered as well. Coarse, dark, curly hair tends to be better camouflage and look thicker than fine, pale hair. Donor plugs of extremely fair-skinned blond or red-haired people may retain a papery-white color that is an unpleasant contrast to surrounding skin tones. (This may not matter for top of the head transplants, but it can be a real problem in the hairline area.)

Age usually is not an important factor. If all other systems are go and the patient still has plenty of healthy hair follicles in the donor areas, it matters little whether he or she is sixteen or seventy-five. A transplant can give her the look of thicker, more attractive hair.

Recent Drugs

A blood pressure-lowering agent called Aldactone (spironolactone) has been found to yield an unexpectedly beneficial side effect. It curbs the activity of the androgens (male hormones) that are responsible for thinning hair in women and men.

Another drug, Minoxidil, is a vasodilator used to control severe hypertension. It is attracting the attention of dermatologists because it results in a universal side effect: hair growth in all patients who receive standard therapeutic doses of the drug. This has led some researchers to consider it a possible topical cure for baldness previously unresponsive to conventional treatment. Minoxidil is believed to act as diuretic that neutralizes male hormones in the scalp and increases the secretion of estrogen.

CHAPTER 13

SPORTS AND YOUR SKIN: PLAYING IT SAFE

Sports: Playing It Safe

Besides being excellent body-shapers, regular exercise and active sports also benefit the skin. As you work out and warm up, the body's natural thermostat dilates tiny capillaries and steps up circulation to cool you off, sending oxygen and moisture to the surface. Sweating, another natural coolant, purges skin of impurities, including oils and salts.

According to studies at the University of California in San Diego, athletes in training have thicker, denser skin than average. One theory is that the internal heat induced by physical exertion spurs the body to produce more collagen. Another study showed that a group of regular exercisers had better skin texture and tone than a matched sample of sedentary people. Under-eye swelling all but disappeared in those who worked out vigorously.

While healthy, vibrant skin is an undeniable dividend of physical activity, your face and body could also wind up badly bruised or abused without proper care. Skin at play is prone to a number of disorders and injuries that may result from sweating, friction, rubbing, abrasion, contact with certain surfaces or equipment, and wearing tight gear. These various traumas sometimes set up very favorable conditions for bacterial, viral, and fungal growth. The result is a higher risk of staph or strep infections, along with complications such as plantar warts and athlete's foot. Dormant or preexisting problems may be intensified as well. Complaints are also environmental, involving exposure to plants and insects, the sun, wind, water, and other elements that relentlessly weather the skin.

Here is a rundown of the more common sports-related syndromes:

Calluses: Probably the most traumatic athletic injury, a callus arises from skin chronically exposed to friction and pressure. The result is a well-defined or circumscribed thickening, actually the body's natural padding formed to protect skin from additional trauma. A callus can grow to considerable size and become less pliant, more painful, and possibly disabling. Unlike a wart (with which it is often confused), it retains normal skin folds and markings and will not show little bleeding points when pared away under local anesthesia.

A callus should be treated only if it is bothersome and interferes with activity; otherwise leave it alone. You risk being sidelined temporarily by surgical procedures. Best approaches are pads to prevent the callus from growing, periodic paring by a dermatologist, and the application of a keratolytic (skin-peeling) agent such as salicylic acid. Some people have underlying foot defects that contribute to callus formation; today these can be corrected with new orthotic devices.

Corns: These are compact calluses frequently found over bony protrusions or defects, erupting from the friction caused by poorly-fitting boots or shoes—hikers and runners beware! The most common variety is the smooth-surfaced, convex hard corn, the favorite residence of which is the fifth or outermost toe.

Soft corns, less common, are painful, moist white masses, which usually crop up within the epidermal tissue between the toes. These, too, can be pared by a dermatologist, peeled away with topical solutions, and prevented by correcting bony defects and wearing properly fitted shoes.

Friction blisters: These are a perennial sports-related nuisance, whether you are handling the ropes while sailing or gripping a racquet. Call them the bane of the weekend athlete who plays his or her sport in concentrated doses without having time to build any protective calluses first. (Experienced athletes often get them at the beginning of a season.) Unlike calluses, blisters arise fairly quickly, forming in response to a sudden, short-lived impact of friction. Cleanse gently, cover with adhesives such as moleskin rather than Band-Aids (which tend to slip), keep feet as dry as possible, and wear a double layer of socks for maximum protection. If you have a big game and can't afford to abandon your sport even temporarily, a doctor can aspirate the blister fluid up to three times during the first twenty-four hours, then cover the lesion with a sterile patch. Or you can try doing it yourself with a sterile needle and gauze dressing.

Jogger's syndrome: Running may result in a curious condition called jogger's nipples—the irritation caused by the rubbing of a runner's shirt against bare skin. Women who jog braless and men are at equal risk, and nipples often turn raw and painful. To prevent this, cover them liberally with petroleum jelly or an adhesive bandage before a long run, or wear a soft-textured T-shirt or sports bra to minimize friction.

Excessive jogging—five or more times a week—may even accelerate the aging process, some experts claim. The natural pull of gravity combined with the constant impact of your feet striking the ground (at a force of about three times your body weight) may jar soft facial tissues and loosen underlying support structures. For this reason, jogging in moderation and horizontal-movement activities such as swimming, hydrocalisthenics (water exercises), and floor and mat routines are considered more desirable.

Jogging in winter may expose the upper lip to extra moisture from a sniffling nose, creating a haven for irritation or infection. Apply a generous coat of chapped-lip ointment or petroleum jelly to help keep the area dry.

Note: Prepare yourself before an extended run with dusting powder, cotton undergarments, and a lightweight outfit with removable layers. These precautions will help avoid irritation, sweating, and overheating, which could aggravate acne or lead to rashes in overly sensitive skin.

Cycling, Riding: Rash Alert: Sitting too long on a saddle may rub, chafe, and irritate the skin because of excessive sweating and heat. To prevent this, wear absorbent cotton underwear and cotton or wool outergarments (avoid synthetic or overly laundered fabrics) and sew extra cloth patches on irritation-prone areas, such as knees and derriere.

Hiking: Wearing tight backpacks and other paraphernalia can result in a case of acne mechanica, which is instigated by constant rubbing and friction (see Chapter 4). And poison ivy, contact dermatitis from tumbleweed, along with insect bites and stings (see below) are natural menaces if you are not properly prepared and protected.

Winter hiking carries a frostbite risk, particularly if weather conditions change unexpectedly. Beware when skin turns from merely pale to white or grayish yellow, and take extra care to protect nose, cheeks, ears, toes, and fingers when you are planning a day in the frosty air. To treat frostbite, increase circulation to the affected area by placing it in warm (not hot) water in a heated environment as quickly as possible. Do not rub with snow or massage vigorously, or you risk damaging delicate tissues. And do not drink alcoholic beverages; these only dilate blood vessels, causing heat to escape.

Sailing, Skiing: A simple, environment-conscious reminder

should suffice here: Protect yourself with a maximum potency sunscreen before any outing, since water and snow will collect and reflect ultraviolet rays, intensifying the damage to your skin. And the wind over sea and slopes will further heighten the effects of solar radiation.

Swimmer's Ear (Otitis Externa): The result of daily immersion over a prolonged period, this infection takes hold in the moist, dark haven of the ear canal and is marked by itching, swelling, pain, tenderness, and sometimes a greenish-yellow discharge. To help prevent it, use cotton ear plugs coated with petroleum jelly to keep out moisture. (Store-bought plugs, with their hard, ridged surfaces, may irritate an already infected ear.) Always dry ears carefully while towelling off, cleanse them regularly and then apply a few drops of Burrow's solution, removing thoroughly after about thirty seconds. For treatment your dermatologist will carefully irrigate the canal with a wick and apply special (usually prescription) drops to fight both the infection and inflammation. Heating pads and aspirin or aspirin substitutes can help ease the pain.

Swimmer's Itch: This condition results from swimming in freshwater lakes that harbor certain parasites. These penetrate the epidermis and induce an allergic reaction, signaled by intense itching and blisters after several days. Calamine lotion and antihistamines will curb the symptoms, along with swimming at the seashore or in a nearby pool!

Tennis, Basketball: Black Toes, Black Heels: Capillaries can take a beating from the constant stop-start pressure as players thrust foward or shift weight with every movement. (Toes are the usual target in tennis, heels in basketball.) Since the vessels leak blood as a result, toes or heels may actually appear black. There is no treatment except staying off your feet until the patchy discolorations disappear. Thick socks and well-fitted shoes are the best preventatives, along with a soft pad in the heel of the sneaker or playing shoe.

Note: Some people are prone to tender, flesh-colored papules on the soles that are actually painful miniature hernias composed of subcutaneous fat. These may disappear spontaneously when the foot is elevated for several hours, only to reappear when a normal position is resumed. The only permanent solution is to avoid all "vertical" sports and switch to those such as swimming and cycling instead.

Turf Burns: These are abrasions in which part of the epidermis (outer skin layer) is actually removed as a result of repeated sliding over rough, unyielding artificial turf. Watch out especially for contact points, such as knees, elbows, and forearms, which take heavy punishment during football, baseball, and soccer. Cleanse the burned area gently with soap and warm water and apply a sterile dressing to help keep it dry and bacteria-free.

Turf Toe: No one is sure why, but this condition, marked by swelling, irritation, and pain, develops when players keep switching between natural to artificial surfaces instead of adapting to one or the other exclusively. Temporarily avoid activity if possible; to prevent turf toe, try working out on one playing field only.

Also watch out for:

Athlete's Foot (not for athletes only): This microscopic plant or fungus roots itself in irritated or lacerated skin between or around the toes and may lie dormant a long time before causing trouble. Excessive sweating resulting from tight footwear, constant friction, infrequent bathing, inadequate ventilation, or all of these is probably the catalyst for the typical outbreak of scaling, itching, inflamed, and blistered skin. If neglected, the condition can lead to severe cracking and fissuring, paving the way for bacterial invasion. Sometimes the nails are affected, too, and marked by thickening and discoloration.

Since athlete's foot sometimes mimics eczema or psoriasis, the wrong remedies may be applied, which can end up making matters worse. Moral: Do not attempt to diagnose or medicate yourself. Adopt these commonsense ways to reduce your risks. Lace sneakers loosely and whenever possible wear open shoes in summer; use wool or cotton socks, not synthetics, and change them often; wash frequently, especially on humid days, followed by a thorough pat-drying (avoid rubbing) and dusting with antifungal powder. Expose skin to a forty-watt incandescent bulb or blow dryer to remove excess moisture.

Antifungal medications in the form of creams or more potent tablets usually can clear up athlete's foot within several weeks. Doctors may also prescribe drying agents, such as Zeasorb powder or other varieties that do not contain talc.

Contact Dermatitis: This common irritation (see Chapter 12) may rear its bothersome head while you are working out in hot, humid weather. It is a special problem for athletes who tape their skin. Sometimes sweating may cause the nickel or other chemicals in a watchband or neckchain to leach out and provoke a reaction. Wear loose, natural-fiber clothing next to sensitive skin, curb moisture by dusting regularly with powder, and cover metal jewelry with a thin coat of clear nail polish to keep chemicals from escaping onto your skin.

Excessive sweating: Overexertion and heavy clothing can cause the body's cooling mechanisms to work overtime, sending excess moisture to the surface. To cut down on the amount you perspire:

Wear lightweight clothing of natural fibers (cotton, linen) when playing vigorously

Shower often, preferably with antibacterial soaps

To curb odor (caused not by sweat but by the bacteria

growing in the warm, moist environment it provides) use antiperspirant sprays containing aluminum compounds

Remove underarm hair to help cut down on bacteria and trapping of moisture

Apply an antiperspirant frequently in hot weather

In rare cases, people troubled by excessive perspiration may have to resort to more drastic measures. For example, a doctor may recommend a saturated solution of aluminum chloride in alcohol applied with a cloth and kept on the affected areas overnight in an airtight wrap.

Ingrown Toenails: The most common cause of this potentially serious complaint, which usually involves the large or great toe, is tight, poorly-fitted shoes, along with inadequate hygiene. Your dermatologist can treat it conservatively by clipping nails down, smoothing out the edges, and packing the clear nail groove with cotton or gauze. Sometimes surgery is indicated.

Insect Bites: Playing outdoors has yet another price: proximity to bees, wasps, hornets, and other painful pests. Some, for example, the honeybee, leave their stingers and venom sacs behind in your skin; others keep their apparatus intact and so can sting repeatedly (take your pick).

The signs are initial pain, often slight, followed by redness, swelling, and itching. Carefully and gently remove any stinger first with a sterile needle or toothpick, since venom will continue to be released by a still-contracting sac for several hours. The best relievers are calamine lotion, ice or cold-water compresses, a paste of water and baking soda, meat tenderizer, and keeping the area elevated. If symptoms are severe and prolonged, see a doctor. Antihistamines or cortisone-based drugs are his usual treatments of choice.

For emergencies, and when a doctor cannot be reached, a new disposable, cigar-shaped device (called Epipen) releases epinephrine, an adrenaline-type drug, to counter serious reactions in allergic individuals (these include difficulty in breathing, lowered blood pressure, and loss of consciousness). Marketed by Center Laboratories, this one-time automatic injector delivers the recommended adult dosage of the drug and has a shelf life of eighteen months.

Prickly Heat (Heat Rash): If you are playing vigorously in humid weather, your body may not be able to release its own cooling moisture quickly enough. So perspiration may get trapped under the skin, resulting in a protest of slightly raised red bumps. The usual targets are the wrists, the bends of elbows and knees, under the breasts, and on the front and sides of the chest. Dust these areas with powder at intervals to quench extra moisture, avoid tight, constricting clothing, and choose cool, shady areas for outdoor recreation whenever possible.

Sports: Watch Your Hair

Hair, literally an extension of skin, can be dry, oily, or a combination of both (oily scalp and brittle, broken ends). Active summer sports call for vigilant sun protection, since ultraviolet rays inflict damage by swelling the outer protective layer (the cuticle) and leaving the inner cortex more exposed. This accelerates moisture loss and alters hair chemistry, causing it to become strawlike and discolored. Not surprisingly, today's conditioners for hair include built-in sunscreens.

Air-conditioned gyms and chlorinated pools are also hair hazards. (Always rinse out chlorinated or salted water immediately after swimming.) To curb dryness and seal splintered ends, coconut or wheat germ oil or petroleum jelly can be applied sparingly during the day and removed at night with a very gentle shampoo or an apple cider/vinegar rinse.

Synthetic Skin for Athletes?

A new soothing "second skin" has been devised to help absorb friction and pressure, ease minor burns, itching, blisters, and abrasions, promote healing, and shield the skin from further irritation or injury. Ninety-six percent water and four percent polyethylene oxide, this elastic, gel-like material absorbs approximately its own weight in water, including blood and perspiration. A temporary "breathable" cover, it can be applied directly over bruised or normal skin and under taping and equipment, where irritation and rubbing are common problems. Developed by Spenco Medical Corporation in Texas, the new synthetic skin is now available in sporting goods and medical supply stores.

References & General Reading

Boughton, Patricia, and Hughes, Martha Ellen. *The Buyer's Guide to Cosmetics*. New York: Random House, 1981.

Conry, Tom. *Consumer's Guide to Cosmetics*. New York: Anchor Press/Doubleday, 1980.

Cunliffe, W. J., M.D., MRCP, and Cotterill, J. A., M.D., MRCP. *The Acnes: Clinical Features, Pathogenesis and Treatment*. London: W. B. Saunders Company Ltd., 1975.

Fitzpatrick, Thomas B., M.D., Ph.D., Arthur Z. Eisen, Klaus Wolff, Irwin M. Freedberg, K. Frank Austen, Eds. *Dermatology in General Medicine*. New York: McGraw Hill Inc., 1979, 1971.

Fulton, James, Jr., M.D., Ph.D., with Hirschorn, Howard H., M.A. *Farewell to Pimples*. Miami, 1977.

Klein, Arnold W., and Sternberg, James H. *The Skin Book*. New York: Macmillan, 1980.

Parrish, John A., M.D., Gilchrest, Barbara, M.D., and Fitzpatrick, Thomas B., M.D. *Between You and Me: A Sensible and Authoritative Guide to the Care and Treatment of Your Skin*. Boston: Little Brown and Company, 1978.

Plewig, Gerd, M.D., and Kligman, Albert, M.D. *Acne: Morphogenesis and Treatment*. Berlin, Heidelberg, New York: Springer-Verlag, 1975.

Schoen, Linda Allen, ed. *The AMA Book of Skin and Hair Care*. Philadelphia, New York: J. B. Lippincott Company, 1976, 1971.

Sutton, Richard L., Jr., M.D., F.R.S. (Edin) and Waisman, Morris, M.D. *York Medical Books*. Dun-Donnelley Publishing Corporation, 1975.

Thiers, Bruce H., M.D., and Dobson, Richard L., M.D. *Yearbook of Dermatology*. Chicago, London: Yearbook Medical Publishers, Inc., 1982.

Zacarian, Setrag A., M.D., F.A.C.P. *Your Skin: Its Problems and Care*. Radnor, Pennsylvania: Chilton Book Company, 1978.

For further information on collagen, contact The Collagen Corporation, Palo Alto, California.

ABOUT THE AUTHORS

Dr. Fredric Haberman is a practicing, board certified dermatologist and skin surgeon in Bergen County, New Jersey, and Manhattan. He is Clinical Instructor of Medicine (Dermatology) at the Albert Einstein College of Medicine and Attending Physician, Department of Medicine (Dermatology), at the Montefiore Hospital Center, both in New York City.

Dr. Haberman is also Vice President of the New Jersey Dermatologic Society, and fellow member of the International Academy of Cosmetic Surgery. He has appeared regularly on many radio and television shows, including *Good Morning New York, Kids Are People Too, Reader's Digest Lifetime* (Cable Health Network), and Storm Field's *Your Body, Your Health*.

Denise Fortino is Health Editor and former Assistant Features Editor at *Harper's Bazaar*. She has written articles on a wide range of subjects for *Harper's* and other national magazines and is currently at work on a book about the art and anguish of being single.

Index

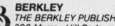